FORENSIC CASEBOOK OF CRIME

John Sanders

TRUE CRIME Library

True Crime Library
A Forum Press Book
by the Paperback Division of
Forum Design,
PO Box 158, London SE20 7QA

An Imprint of True Crime Library
© 2000 Forum Design
© 2000 John Sanders
All rights reserved

Designed and typeset by Ben James
Printed and bound in Great Britain by
Cox & Wyman, Reading, Berkshire

ISBN 1-874358-36-2

For M

CONTENTS

1

THE CORPSE THAT CRIED

"Slow pulsation was now observed in the neck,"
wrote Dr. Benstead. "And it became apparent that
the 'body' was just breathing"

Kim Nevitt had no idea where she was. She was awake, she knew that, and she wasn't alone. She could see that between the bed on which she lay and the bright light on the ceiling was imposed the head of a pretty young nurse. And there was a heavy smell of antiseptic in the air.

"You've been on TV and in all the papers," the nurse smiled at her. Then she added in rather a matter-of-fact way, "You've been dead, you know."

"You've been dead!"

It didn't mean much to Mrs. Nevitt at that moment. She felt very weak and her mouth was sore from the tubes that had been forced down her throat as conduits. All she wanted to do was sleep. She was to learn the full extraordinary story later.

It began early in the morning of Friday, 31st October, 1969, when two council workmen driving their sand lorry over the beach at Waterloo, near Liverpool, found the body of a woman. The workmen called the police, who in turn called a doctor. Just after nine o'clock the doctor, deciding that the body was not breathing and there was no pulse, certified the woman was dead.

Her body was covered with loose tarpaulins, and the Home Office forensic pathologist, Dr. John Benstead, was summoned from his home at Southport.

While Dr. Benstead was on his way the police, suspecting they had a murder case on their hands, formed a task force and began to search the beach for clues. After all, there were fresh tyre-marks by the body, probably made by the vehicle used by the assailants either to attack the woman or to dump her where she was found. That these were in fact the tyre-marks of the council workmen's sand lorry had not, it seems, registered for the moment.

An hour later Dr. Benstead arrived. The tarpaulins were lifted, and crouching down on the beach alongside the body he began a cursory examination. The woman was in her early twenties, fresh-faced and neatly dressed.

He sensed at once that something was very unusual about this body. "There was no dew on the corpse," he wrote later in his case notes. "Nor were there any obvious signs of violence." He also noted that rigor mortis was not present, nor was there any hypostasis (post-mortem lividity). When a person dies there is a complete muscular relaxation which is then followed by a stiffening of the muscular systems – rigor mortis. The process begins with the eyelids and descends down through the entire body over a period generally of about 12 hours. It is not, contrary to popular belief, a reliable way of determining time of death, because the time it takes varies with local conditions. Dr. Benstead also noted the body temperature was 27.2 degrees Centigrade. "It was obvious that these findings were inconsistent with the information I had been given – that the woman was certified as dead by the police doctor who had seen her an hour or so earlier. I decided that his thermometer needed checking – or even perhaps that mine did. So I sent an officer to find out what kind of thermometer the police doctor used and at what part of the body the reading had been taken."

Benstead was definitely puzzled. Of the three cardinal signs of death, algor (cooling), rigor (stiffening) and livor (staining), he could see only algor. Rigor was still absent, and livor, or hypostasis, couldn't be properly assessed in that exposed part of the beach without removing the woman's clothing. "As far as I'm concerned she isn't dead yet," he told a police officer. He ordered the body to be taken to Waterloo mortuary for a detailed post-mortem examination, and followed the police there in his red sports car.

In the mortuary the body was placed on a slab and again Dr. Benstead bent over it. The woman's features were still fresh-coloured; prising open her mouth, he found fresh saliva. Somehow he was convinced she was just alive, although to all intents and purposes that did not seem possible. Then as he stood up, looking intently at the corpse, he saw a tiny tear trickle out of one of its eyes and roll down its cheek.

"Slow pulsation was now observed in the neck," he wrote. "And it became apparent that the 'body' was just breathing."

A police officer standing by the pathologist's side was rather less restrained. He yelled out, "She's alive!" – and an urgent flurry of activity engulfed the mortuary. Policemen ripped off their coats and placed them under and around the woman; her limbs were chafed, and an ambulance was called. When it arrived hot-water bottles were pressed around her, and intermittent oxygen was given. Benstead jumped into the ambulance with his patient and travelled to Walton Hospital with her. She was attended to immediately, but there was now no sign of life. Was she drugged, or was she suffering deeply from hypothermia, the doctors wondered as they wired her up to an ECG machine. Still the life response was negative. Then, once again, came a flicker of life.

Just how tiny that flicker was can be gauged from the temperature readings on the woman. In the mortuary Dr. Benstead had noted her temperature at 26 degrees Centigrade (78 Fahrenheit). Half an hour later, in the hospital, the reading was 25 degrees Centigrade (77 Fahrenheit). Seven hours after admission her temperature had dropped to 24 degrees Centigrade (75 Fahrenheit). But of two things there was no doubt – she was alive, even if only just, and she owed her life to the keen observation of the pathologist John Benstead, who next day was making headlines as the "Teardrop Hero."

Over the next few hours clues began to emerge about the woman. Her name was Kim Nevitt, she was married, had children, and lived in Liverpool. When she was given a stomach wash Benstead noted that it revealed 13 milligrams of Tuinal, a barbiturate drug. "Twenty-three capsules of unknown strength were probably available to her," he calculated. He also reckoned that she must have arrived on the beach at about one o'clock in the morning, which meant that she lay there for seven hours before the two council workmen found her. The maximum temperature in Liverpool that night did not reach 12 degrees Centigrade and there had been a keen easterly wind. All in all, Kim Nevitt was a patient who was extremely lucky to be alive.

For the next 72 hours she remained unconscious and her life hung in the balance. She was kept in intensive care while the medical staff at Walton Hospital slowly brought her temperature up to normal from the 26 degrees Centigrade (78 degrees Fahrenheit) it had been in the mortuary. When she recovered consciousness a doctor explained to Kim later that if she had stayed in bed in her flat the overdose would certainly have killed her. But because her body became so cold on the beach her blood circulation slowed down, and the barbiturate stayed in her stomach instead of circulating around her body.

She had effectively been frozen alive, suspended in a deep hypothermia, a condition in which there are no visible signs of life such as breathing or heartbeat. Dr. Benstead wrote, "She probably passed from barbiturate coma with hypothermia into true hypothermic stupor, as is likely to happen in many cases of barbiturate poisoning where the victim is not rescued." She entered into a state where she would be mistaken for dead probably between 2.15 and 4.45 a.m. Had she died, the cause would undoubtedly have been from hypothermia and/or broncho-pneumonia rather than from any lethal concentration of poison still present in the body.

As Kim recovered her strength she was able to show visitors the mortuary tag which was on her wrist when she arrived at the hospital, and which she was allowed to keep. It said, "Dead on arrival – name unknown." One of her visitors was Dr. Benstead, who remarked, "You're looking a lot better than when I last saw you."

A week after admission Kim was well enough to leave hospital, and she made a full recovery. The story she told was sadly familiar. She was 23, and her marriage had broken up. Her three children, all girls aged nine, six and five, were in the care of the local authority.

For months she had been working as a clerk during the day and a waitress at night, trying to save enough money to get a home together for herself and her children. She alternated between being depressed just by thinking of the future and hoping that if she could make enough money everything would be all right.

That October night the depression was winning. The children had been away for 12 months, and to make matters worse Kim had recently suffered a debilitating kidney infection. She was listening to the radio when she decided quite suddenly to kill herself. She lay on her bed, took a nearly full box of barbiturates, pushing the pills into her mouth and swallowing them, and then tried to get some sleep.

But before the pills took effect she made up her mind that she didn't want to die in a dingy bed-sit. She would go down to the beach at Seaforth to breathe in some good salt air for the last time.

So at one o'clock in the morning she put on her pink overall and best fawn coat with a fur collar and began to walk the half-mile or so to the beach. She vaguely remembered being on the beach, and then stumbling. She said afterwards that she was conscious of having a terrible nightmare, and of desperately wanting someone to wake her up from it.

Kim's story had a happy ending. After she left hospital she was looked after by friends, then she found a flat of her own and went back to work. A year later she had saved enough money to set up home in a quiet Liverpool suburb and buy enough furniture to have her children with her. Two years after being given up for dead she was able to say, "I feel I've never been happier, and I have so much to look forward to."

After it was all over Dr. Benstead observed with the characteristic diligence of a skilled forensic pathologist:

"This incident illustrates how excessively careful should be the certification of death in any circumstances where a body has not been under continuous surveillance for a reasonable time, particularly where only a limited examination is permitted or possible. Even at the hospital, had the staff not been alerted, this patient might well have been certified dead for a second time. She would then have been neatly filed away in a refrigerator and her case report would never have been written. Unless there is obvious rigor and hypostasis, quite apart from cooling, continuous assessment or at least re-examination after an appropriate interval is always advisable."

The Kim Nevitt case excited a flurry of political and medical comment, for although other corpses have since "come alive" in the mortuary, hers was the first recorded case. Although the Home Office made it clear that Mrs Nevitt owed her life to the "thoroughness with which the pathologist carried out his duties," MPs asked for detailed reports, implying in some instances, much to Benstead's fury, that he had been in error in first sending the body to a mortuary and not straight to hospital. One of the areas of anxiety concerned possible transplant donors, although Benstead assured MPs that donors were always under continuous medical attention for some time before they died, so that a mistake was impossible. Medical papers were written on the case, particularly on the methodology of establishing time of death, often so vital a piece of evidence in murder cases. Dr. Benstead wrote to an inquiring professor of medicine, "The real problem is where one gives wide limits with customary caution but in an endeavour to be helpful produces a probability which is then regarded by everyone but the unhappy pathologist as an accurate deduction." He sometimes got it wrong himself, he said, adding, "Just at the moment my name is mud in the city of Manchester because a time-of-death estimate of mine was wildly out. Fortunately no charge resulted."

Dr. Benstead was never to forget Kim Nevitt – he used to say he wasn't going to let anyone else forget her, either. Although he twice announced the body alive while others were convinced she was dead, he was several times wrongly reported as "that pathologist who pronounced Kim Nevitt dead when she was still alive." Later Kim Nevitt sold her story to a Sunday newspaper. "She was well paid for it too," Benstead recalled. "But when I went to be paid for my work I was told I was getting nothing because I had had nothing to do!" In a veiled reference to Kim's newspaper windfall, he reported to Lancashire CID, "I would like to express my deep admiration of the resuscitation team at Walton Hospital and my gratification that Mrs. Nevitt appears to have suffered no ill effects – and indeed may even be better off after her extraordinary experience."

The jokes aside, the medical world fortunately did not forget Kim Nevitt either. A few years later a young Lancashire doctor was found slumped over the wheel of his car parked in a wood near Castleton, Derbyshire. At first the police physician called to the case thought the victim was dead, because there was no heartbeat or pulse. But remembering Kim Nevitt, he decided to make a second check. He noted that the spot was cold and the body temperature was low. The young doctor was transferred from the mortuary where he had been taken to Sheffield Royal Hospital, where electronic tests detected faint heart movement. For the next six hours the medical staff fought to try to save his life, but to no avail.

Nor, incidentally, did Kim Nevitt ever forget John Benstead and the way he restored her to life and happiness. When the pathologist died many years later she went to his funeral, remarking that it could so easily have been the other way around – he could have been a mourner at hers.

The idea that any of us might be certified dead while we are still alive, and that we might wake up in a mortuary, an undertaker's parlour or a crematorium, is a haunting one. But it has happened. In 1969 the relatives of a Yorkshire man who was gravely ill were told that his death was imminent. A male nurse told the man's wife that when her husband died she should send for an undertaker and next day call on the doctor for a death certificate. Shortly afterwards the man lapsed into a coma, and his wife thought he had died. She called the undertaker, who noticed signs of breathing only after he had removed the body to his premises. The man was rushed to hospital but survived only a few hours. It was established that he was moribund when he was removed by the undertaker, and that fortunately the premature removal had not accelerated his death.

In another incident, in 1950, a woman aged 75 was brought into a London hospital having been found, some 20 minutes previously, lying on common ground cold and apparently lifeless. As the ambulance arrived with her body at the casualty department a doctor was summoned to it. He placed a hand on her chest and felt for her pulse, and unable to find it pronounced her dead. The woman was taken to the mortuary, stripped and laid on a slab. Some four or five minutes afterwards she began to breathe visibly. She was examined by stethoscope, which revealed a heart-beat. She survived for another two and a quarter hours.

So the first thing that the forensic pathologist must decide when he starts to examine a corpse is whether or not it really is a corpse, or a person unconscious. Easy enough, you may think, but cases are known in which people suffering from concussion, electrocution, exposure, grave shock or severe illness have been pronounced dead just because they are not moving, because there have been no outward signs of breathing, or because the surface of the body is cold. In cases of drowning particularly, it is often difficult to decide whether the victim has died. People pulled unconscious from the water are often cold and stiff. One or two hours may pass before signs of life appear. In one case on record the victim was not restored until resuscitation techniques had been applied for eight and a half hours. In other cases pathologists have noted nothing more than "a lingering vitality" about a body which has been subsequently resuscitated. But if the drowned adult has been under water for more than half an hour there is obviously no hope of resuscitation.

Similarly there can be no hope for someone found hanging when the body is cold and rigid. When execution by hanging was the rule in Britain before 1965 the body of the prisoner was always certified dead immediately after execution. The cause of death was habitually given as a broken neck. Even so, the prisoner was always left hanging below the trap-door of the scaffold for an hour. No hangman who has written his memoirs – and there have been plenty of them – has explained why the body was left hanging, and the irresistible inference must be that medical opinion suspected that even after pronouncing "death" there was always the faintest chance that the hanged man could be resuscitated.

Electrocution is another case where pronouncement of death is not always easy. An electrocuted body can look positively dead, but there are many cases on record of lives saved in electrocution cases by continuing artificial respiration for long periods. As electrocution has been widely used in America as a means of execution, the question has to be asked: could any executed prisoner have been resuscitated if the current had been switched off at any given time before the execution was completed?

The question has to be asked too as to what might have happened to Kim Nevitt if Dr. Benstead had not discovered that she was alive? The spectre of being buried while you are still alive is a grotesque one – but is it possible? The answer is no, it is not. There is no authenticated case on record in the UK of premature burial, and the way the law stands no such thing could actually happen, despite near-misses like Kim Nevitt. One authority who collected examples of premature burial across the world and across the centuries came up with 46 cases – but none of them stand up to scientific scrutiny. The fear has always been greater than the reality, and has provided great scope for fertile imagination, as witness this report in *The Lancet* in 1900:

"Shortly after the great cholera visitation of 1866 Dr. Filipp Pacini, professor of anatomy in Florence, called attention to the subject [of being buried while still alive]. He cited not a few cases in which the patient, certified dead, had come to life on his way to the cemetery, and he started the not unnatural, if horrible, inference, that the resuscitation referred to may in several instances have come about within the grave itself. To such an extent has this fear of premature burial been carried in America that an association, called the American Society for the Prevention of Premature Burial, was actually started there."

The safeguards that are in position in Britain are that the cause of death must be certified, and a dead body cannot be buried or cremated without the certificate of the registrar or an order of a coroner. A GP who signs a death certificate, though, can theoretically do so without seeing or examining the body, which is where there is always a slight chance of initial error or irregular practice. In one case a doctor gave a death certificate for an "old lady" he had been attending in a large three-storey house converted into apartments. A girl who also lived in the house had called at the doctor's surgery and reported, "The old lady's dead." What neither she nor the doctor knew was that there were two old ladies living in the house. The girl was reporting the death of her grandmother who lived at the top of the house, but the doctor assumed her to mean the "old lady" who lived on the second floor and was one of his patients. Without further inquiry he issued a death certificate for his patient, who was still very much alive. The mistake was swiftly corrected.

Today a certifying GP must state on the certificate whether he saw the body after death, and how long before death he last saw the dead person alive. If he says he has not seen the body after death, or that he has not attended the dead person within two weeks before death, the registrar will refer the case to the coroner for investigation.

The story of Kim Nevitt was an episode in Dr. Benstead's career which unusually had a happy ending. For as is the lot of pathologists and forensic scientists, death was a way of life for 30 years for the Exeter-born doctor – death in its grimmest aspect, sudden, often violent, and invariably nasty. As a Home Office pathologist based in Southport, he spent a lifetime involved in investigating murder, suicide and horrifying accidents.

John Benstead was a dapper, slightly eccentric figure. He generally wore a bow tie and frequently sported a carnation in his buttonhole. He had a schoolboyish love of trains that ran to a complex toy railway set-up in his own home, and he drove a red sports car from one morgue to another. He could let rip at slackness using language that made officials blanch. In his report to the Home Office on the "resurrection" of Kim Nevitt he wrote, "Further examination of the body was seriously delayed by the absence of a mortuary attendant attached to the squalid and windswept shed designated with sardonic humour as a mortuary by a local authority whose cynically indifferent incompetence in this sphere is a constant source of irritation and anxiety to Home

Office and other pathologists." He could be brutally candid too with any colleague he thought was stuffy. Once when he was talking to a psychiatrist in company with a couple of doctors about mental illness the psychiatrist began to talk about "a compulsorily detained psychiatric patient." Benstead interrupted, "Excuse me, do you mean a nutter?"

Throughout his colourful career Benstead remained a warm, humorous man with a nice line in self-deprecation. On his desk was a framed letter of rebuke from the local area health authority, a body with which he had had some spiky exchanges. "It's there because it amuses me," he would tell inquirers. The words complained of might themselves have been framed and put on exhibit. Benstead had written:

"Despite repeated requests by coroners, by police and by pathologists, and in contrast to the generally satisfactory conditions within the county boroughs, the Lancashire County authority in its approach to mortuary matters must be quite particularly backward even when considered only by the standards of previous centuries. In this decade [this was in the 1960s] I have conducted a post-mortem in a murder case where a constable held a bulb on a flex towards a primitive slab in an outhouse where, without any assistance, I made an examination which led to the execution of the accused."

Benstead thought that Parliament had done the nation no favours when hanging was abolished in 1965. He once said that that decision effectively abolished murder itself. "For make no mistake, it was the unique punishment which singled out murder as such a reprehensible crime from other felonies and from lesser homicides." So-called life imprisonment and the defence of diminished responsibility had taken much of the sting from pathologists' evidence in murder trials, and shifted the emphasis perhaps to the psychiatrists, "who these days all seem to agree with each other." Other crimes in terms of the punishment meted out for them were now the equal of murder, or sometimes even greater than murder, which had been reduced to "the status of an accident within an incident, or if you like an incident within an accident." He was pro-abortion too – thankful, he said, that since the Act legitimising abortion he had seen only one fatal criminal abortion.

John Benstead's father wanted him to be a lawyer, but medicine quickly became an interest, and with it specialist medicine. After graduation he went on a trip across the world as a young married man, investigating a government plan to market whale meat for feeding a population deprived of protein by wartime rationing. He sampled the whale meat himself, and reported that fresh whale steaks were really quite palatable. The problem, though, was in preserving them, so the doubtful pleasure of whale meat was spared the British public.

Back in England, Benstead lectured at Leeds in pathology and joined the pathological team based at Southport, where he developed an interest in forensic medicine. He was quickly appointed as an acting Home Office pathologist, later taking over the position permanently.

In his first case Benstead had to deal with a mother who had fixed up a room with a gas pipe to kill herself and her children. "Officially she committed a murder," he recalled. "But for me such cases are really human tragedies."

He was involved in numerous cases which started out as suspected murder investigations, but became something quite different once he started working on them. One typical incident was a railway case in which a train driver at Warrington was found dead in his cab with suspicious head injuries. Benstead found a piece of projecting metal on a wall, and was able to show that the driver leaning out of his cab might well have hit it. The metal projection was taken down and its surface was analysed in a laboratory, where traces of flesh on the metal confirmed his deduction.

For a pathologist confronted with a corpse the manner of death is not always obvious, and he must be constantly on his guard. In 1972 Benstead was called into a case in which the victim was found in bed stabbed with a knife. A crime of passion? Far from it. During the post-mortem he revealed that before the stabbing the victim had been electrocuted by the killer. In another case a young boy was found dead and hanging in a way indicative of some sort of game or experiment that had gone wrong. The sophisticated killer had supplied some extra wounds to the victim, wounds which were clearly meant to put the pathologist off the scent. In fact Benstead proved that the young boy had been strangled by the killer.

"These are the kind of bizarre cases that keep one constantly on the alert," Benstead said. With characteristic candour he admitted that he may not have always been right. "There are about half a dozen post-mortems that I would love to do again if only it were possible."

After the Kim Nevitt case Benstead was back in the headlines again during the hunt for the Yorkshire Ripper. The body of 26-year-old prostitute Joan Harrison had been discovered on waste land at Preston, and due to the cruel work of a Sunderland hoaxer who deliberately misled detectives it was thought that she might be another victim of the Ripper.

But Benstead was unconvinced. "There are certain dissimilarities that make me think this is not the Ripper," he wrote in his case notes. And so it proved to be, when the Yorkshire Ripper, Peter Sutcliffe, later disclaimed responsibility for the murder. The case remained unsolved, but the pathologist never gave up hope of seeing the file satisfactorily closed on every murder he handled. He took heart from cases like that of a 17-year-old St Helens girl, Janet Cheetham, who was found dead in an alleyway near her home in December, 1981.

Janet, who had alighted from a bus at 11.20 on a snowy night after a night out with friends, was attacked so ferociously that Benstead at first thought the injuries were consistent with the work of two men. He said she must have put up a tremendous fight, concluding that she died from asphyxia and shock caused by multiple injuries and strangulation with an army scarf left at the scene of the crime. There were few clues and none of any value, and the case looked as if it would lie for ever in the unsolved file. But four years later, in October 1985, 20 year-old supermarket supervisor Andrew Brent confessed to killing Janet.

Brent was only just 16 at the time, an army cadet with an ambition to go to Sandhurst. He had got off the bus with Janet and talked to her. There was some sexual contact, and she hit him. They fought, and during the fight she suffered a severe head injury. Brent said he thought she was going to die, and tried to quicken the event by strangling her. He then left her for dead. Next day he helped his mother in her cafe to serve coffee to scene-of-crime officers investigating the murder.

Besides being a keen army cadet, Andrew Brent was a football referee. He had left his cadet scarf at the murder scene, and dropped his football referee's whistle there too, but a connection between the two was never established. Dr. Benstead watched him as he was sentenced at Liverpool Crown Court to life imprisonment in February, 1986. It had taken four years, but another murder file was finally closed.

2

HOW FIGHTING JAMES KELLY DIED

The only career left to him was one of social revenge—a career manifested in drunkenness, street brawling and bashing policemen

John Benstead freely confessed he wasn't always right. But on one of the controversial post-mortems he conducted he stood four-square behind his findings. This was on James Kelly, a 53-year-old unemployed bachelor who lived with his mother in Sleaford Road, Huyton. A violent drunk, Kelly died in the sort of circumstances that frequently send a shudder of apprehension and alarm across the land – he died in police custody.

If ever a man was fated to be one of life's losers, such a man was James Kelly. At school he was slow at his lessons and unable to learn the simplest things. For this he was taunted by fellow-pupils, and left school disillusioned and almost illiterate. Called up as a National Serviceman, he proved too hopeless even for that man's army, and was discharged as "mentally deficient, dull and backward." His discharge certificate, dated January 1947, drew attention to a burgeoning criminal record, which included a jail sentence when he was sixteen, adding, "He had difficulty in adjusting to the Pioneer Corps and although liking labouring cannot adjust to his fellow soldiers or to discipline."

His short army career recorded two dozen minor offences, mostly for absence without leave. His illiteracy, said the report, cut him off from his own home, which contributed to his depression – "he controls his aggressive feelings with difficulty." Thus James Kelly, failed soldier, was ejected from the ranks of the Pioneer Corps back into civvy street. He was short and muscular with a considerable ability to absorb alcohol, and thereby ideally suited for the only career left to him – one of anti-social revenge on life which had turned its back on him, a career manifested in drunkenness, street brawling, and bashing policemen.

For the first four years after his army discharge Kelly simmered silently. Then, in the 21 years between 1953 and 1974, the year of his death, the civilian record states that he was convicted on 12 separate occasions of minor offences relating to drunkenness and violence, including two assaults on police officers. If during this time Kelly maintained some semblance of the man of muscle he liked to think he was, internally he was in a sorry state. Ravaged by drink and fighting, he was suffering from enlargement of the heart, high blood-pressure and obesity. He had become increasingly short of breath and any exertion triggered off violent chest pains. Examined at Broadgreen Hospital five years before his death, he was diagnosed as having angina pectoris, a condition resulting from the inability of the heart muscle to obtain sufficient oxygen via the blood for its proper function, especially when the heart is stressed by excitement or exertion. Angina pectoris frequently leads to a disease called atheroma – or in its most severe form, atherosclerosis. This is a serious disorder which blocks one or both of the coronary arteries – it has a well-recognised liability to produce sudden death. In the early 1970s the average time of survival following diagnosis was between eight to ten years, but the condition could be adversely affected by enlargement of the heart, high blood-pressure, and obesity, from all of which Kelly suffered. So it was that every time James Kelly took a drink, and squared up to the next man at the bar, he was effectively playing Russian roulette.

Two days before he died Kelly went to hospital for a check-up. He considered such visits a waste of time, and sometimes never turned up after an appointment was booked. This time he pooh-poohed the anxious looks of the doctors and nurses and tried to convince them he was vastly improved. "I can walk half a mile on the level without bringing on any chest pains now," he boasted. But a doctor noted that the simple effort of climbing on to the examination couch made Kelly breathless, and wrote on his notes, "He is in mild heart failure."

That was on June 18th, 1979, and two days later, on Wednesday, June 20th, Kelly woke up with something to celebrate, although of course he did not need something to celebrate in order to take a walk to the pub. His brother William was home from Australia, so at 7.30 p.m. the two men settled down at the Oak Tree pub and stayed there until shortly after closing time. William Kelly recalled that each of them drank six or seven pints of beer and a couple of whiskies.

At around 10.45 William walked off to look for a taxi, leaving brother James standing outside the pub chatting to a friend. James was thought to be sober and quite capable of making his way home, a ten to fifteen minute walk. But for the next hour and a quarter he disappeared – it proved impossible to trace his movements. All that is known is that at 11.20 p.m., during this missing period, an anonymous 999 caller reported that a man was being badly beaten up outside the Eagle and Child pub, in the same general area as the Oak Tree. But when police arrived at the scene they could find no disturbance.

Just before midnight, more than a full hour after he was last seen outside the Oak Tree, then just six or seven minutes' walk away, Kelly "reappeared" in Barkbeth Road, which was on his normal way home. He was singing and shouting on a patch of waste land, and he was clearly very drunk. One observer said he was "rolling around," another that he was "lying on his back with his legs in the air." Kelly tried to get up from the ground but fell over again. Two teenage boys approached him and asked him if he needed help; Kelly's extremely abusive reply sent them running off to fetch assistance. They flagged down a police car, but PCs Frederick Browning and Robert Evans had already had the situation reported to them by another passer-by, and now they drove fast to the incident scene.

With their headlights fully on, the officers drove on to the waste land and saw Kelly either sitting or kneeling on the ground. What happened next was disputed. Five witnesses, together with the two policemen, said that Kelly grabbed the front of the police car and tried either to haul himself upright on it or actually to push the car bodily backwards, but he only succeeded in falling over again. But another witness said that the police car struck Kelly twice, knocking him to the ground on both occasions. Later, however, the same witness retracted that statement and said that "the car drove very slowly, then more or less stopped and touched him at the same time," whereupon Kelly fell over. Another witness said that the police car "just touched" Kelly, causing him to fall to the ground.

In front of a growing group of people, Browning and Evans next tried to arrest Kelly. PC Evans said Kelly swore at him and attacked him, striking him about the face and body. There was a violent struggle, and both men fell to the ground. Evans said that he struck Kelly several times with his fists, purely in self-defence. Browning then left the car and held Kelly's legs. They got Kelly to his feet and attempted to push him into their car through the nearside door, but the drunken man fought like a tiger. During the struggle Evans saw Kelly move his hand to a bottle in his pocket. The police officer shouted to Browning, who took the bottle, half-full of whisky, from Kelly, opened the car boot, placed it inside and then went back to help his colleague.

The officers were now faced with the problem of getting the struggling Kelly into their car, a two-door Ford Escort. PC Evans admitted later that he squeezed the drunk's testicles in order to encourage him to get in and that this proved effective, at least for a few seconds. "Somehow or other," said Evans, "Kelly got across the car and either fell out or got out of the opposite door." Evans went round the car and again closed with Kelly, and the two of them struggled until they were both exhausted. During this part of the fracas PC Browning stood or knelt on Kelly's feet. Browning said he saw Kelly bite PC Evans, who cried out and punched the drunk.

Three teenage brothers watching the disturbance substantially agreed with the police officers' account of what happened; all three of them felt that the two policemen did no more than restrain Kelly, who was struggling violently and kicking out all through the episode. Another witness, however, said that when the policemen first approached Kelly it was PC Evans who struck the first blows, hitting the drunk once or twice on the upper part of his body and possibly in the face with his fist. Only after this, said the witness, did Kelly begin to hit back. The witness added that PC Evans hit Kelly three or four more times while he was on the ground. The witness's wife heard Kelly shout, "Man to man, you bastards," and PC Evans's reply, "Do you want another one?"

Some of the witnesses whose evidence suggested that the police over-reacted made statements which appeared to be unreliable. Two of them assumed that when PC Evans went to the boot of the car and opened it he took out a weapon, but neither of them saw what it was. Another witness said that when Kelly was on the ground, after he had emerged from the car he was struck three or four times with a truncheon by PC Browning. But five days after making that statement the witness amended it to say that he saw "the officer's right arm going up and down three or four times with a clubbing motion in the direction of the man on the ground," but he did not actually see the truncheon. The wife of that witness never saw Kelly "doing anything wrong," and never heard him make a sound. PC Browning, she said, "kicked hell out of Kelly."

A young man watching what was going on from the thirteenth floor of a nearby block of flats said that when the officers first approached Kelly and led him to the car they acted in "a friendly manner." However, at the car Kelly went down, and both officers began punching him as he lay on the ground. Then after one of the policemen had gone to the boot of the car he began to club Kelly, although the observer saw no weapon in his hand – there was a noise "like two blocks of wood being knocked together." This witness, like several others, thought that when Kelly was put in the car on one side he was pulled out on the other side. "Kelly was then given another going over, although this time it wasn't so bad, they were more throwing him around." Later the same witness admitted that his attention was distracted for two short periods and he hadn't actually seen Kelly emerging from the car – he returned to see him lying on his side on the ground outside the car with the policemen merely "standing over him."

A young woman who thought Kelly was dragged out of the car admitted she couldn't see properly. In a later statement she made no mention of Kelly being dragged from the car, and she specifically stated that at no time did she "see either policeman do anything to the man."

The arrival of the police van with the two reinforcements did not deter Kelly. One of the new arrivals said Kelly was making a roaring noise but no words were distinguishable. As he approached Kelly he received a painful kick on the knee, and endeavoured to handcuff the drunk, who was "struggling like a madman." He managed to handcuff Kelly's free wrist but couldn't handcuff the other wrist even when his colleagues tried to help, and he was hit several times by Kelly's free arm, one blow cracking a tooth. Still shouting, kicking out to right and left, and "struggling furiously," Kelly was finally handcuffed and lifted bodily into the van. Even then he continued to lash out with his feet and to shout abuse. PC Evans, who got into the van with him, couldn't understand what he was saying, and Browning thought the prisoner was "mumbling."

It was at this stage that the recollection of the four policemen differed in detail. Was Kelly struggling in the van or was he reasonably still? Were his words audible, or was he talking gibberish? One officer said that Kelly neither moved nor spoke during the journey to Huyton police station. In the event, he clearly must have been more subdued, constrained by the small area of the van and the handcuffs. The journey took five minutes, and when they arrived two other policemen were waiting to assist them. They tried to lift Kelly out of the van, but the prisoner proved heavier than they imagined, and slipped through their hands, falling heavily on the ground. From there he was carried up the four steps to the charge office and laid on his back on the floor. As he was brought from the darkness of the yard into the light of the office the officers saw that he was unconscious and making no sound or movement. One officer felt for the prisoner's pulse and listened for his heart-beat but heard nothing. Kelly's face meanwhile was becoming a deepening blue. Almost certainly at this point he was already dead, having died either in the van or as he was being carried out of it.

The officers applied heart massage and called for an ambulance, which astonishingly arrived between sixty and ninety seconds. The ambulance-men also tried heart massage – a couple of hefty blows over the sternum – but Kelly didn't respond. Only seven minutes later, immediately upon his arrival at the hospital, he was certified dead by the casualty doctor, who like the ambulance-men noticed no particular marks on the body.

Next day inquiries were immediately set in motion, for the death of a man in police custody, even a raving drunk like James Kelly, causes eyebrows to rise in a Western democratised country, and no one is entirely satisfied until the preceding events are gone over in detail and every effort is made to establish the truth of what happened. The coroner as soon as he was informed instructed John Benstead to begin a post-mortem. All that Benstead was told when he arrived at Whiston Hospital mortuary was that the dead man had been arrested for being drunk and disorderly, that he had been extremely violent, and was seen to go blue in the face and collapse when he arrived at the police station. He also heard that two of the officers involved were off duty with slight injuries.

In this case, Benstead noted at once, Kelly was

undoubtedly dead. Rigor mortis was fully developed, and dark hypostasis was present on the back of the corpse. There were some tattoo marks, a few old scars on the scalp and a wart on the back.

Benstead listed twenty-three "recent marks" – grazes and small bruises, all of no importance, and some others which were even more trivial. Injuries number six and seven were a half-inch graze on the gums in the centre of the mouth and a half-inch graze on the chin. These two injuries were to loom large in a subsequent investigation.

He removed the heart for microscopic examination later, noting that "the left ventricle was much thickened and there was a patch of dense fibrosis half an inch thick in the posterior wall. The right ventricle showed an unusual excess of covering and infiltrating fat; the smaller coronary arteries were extremely narrow." But some sixth sense, vital to a forensic pathologist, prompted him to proceed cautiously. He indicated in a general way that he thought death was due to heart failure, but decided to reserve his opinion about the exact cause. What concerned him were the injuries on Kelly's body; small and insignificant though they were, they might just be hiding something.

If Benstead's general assumption was correct and it was all down to Kelly's heart, the part played by alcohol may be judged from the fact that a sample he took from the dead man showed a blood alcohol level of 331 milligrams% – that is, 331 milligrams of alcohol per 100 mls of blood. As a yardstick to measure this by, the drink-driving alcohol limit is currently 80 milligrams. To achieve his level Kelly must have drunk at least 200 grams of alcohol, that is, thirteen and a half pints of beer or 26 single whiskies. But this theoretical maximum peak is calculated on the basis of the alcohol being consumed in one dose and instantly absorbed – a condition never fulfilled in practice and certainly not in Kelly's case, where drinking was said to have happened over about two and a half hours. So in order to produce a peak of 331 milligrams per cent Kelly's intake would need to be increased by about a third as much again, that is to about 18 pints 16 double whiskies.

Given those figures, the evidence of William Kelly, the brother home from Australia who was James Kelly's sole drinking companion that night, was remarkable. James, William told the police, "seldom went out for a drink." If this seems astonishing, it should be remembered that William had been away for some time, and that he might have been judging his older brother by his own personal standards. Even so, it was in marked contrast to Kelly's criminal record. It is doubtful whether many men not in regular drinking practice could down "six pints of beer and a couple of whiskies" (William's estimate of James Kelly's intake during their meeting) in a single session and remain sober; it is equally doubtful if they could ever consume enough drink to achieve a blood alcohol of 331 mgs. per cent. It follows, though, that if William was right, and lack of cash due to his unemployment had caused Kelly to abstain for some time, then the effect of a suddenly raised blood alcohol would be all the greater for his being unaccustomed to it.

But always supposing that William Kelly was right in his assessment of what he and his brother drank at the Oak Tree that night, where did James Kelly get the difference between six pints and a couple of whiskies and 18 pints or 16doubles in the hour and a quarter after he was last seen chatting to a friend outside the Oak Tree and his sighting on the waste land at Barkbeth Road? Could he have drunk 12 more pints or 14 more doubles in so short a time? When he left the Oak Tree he seemed to be sober – so said his friend, and so said the landlord, too. The landlord also said that half-bottles of whisky such as the police found in Kelly's pocket were not sold at the Oak Tree. William Kelly was certain that his brother couldn't have bought any extra drink, because James didn't have a penny on him when he left the pub.

Benstead decided that there were three possible answers to the conundrum. The first was that Kelly could have been drinking all day, and thus went into the evening session with an already elevated blood alcohol. Against this was the evidence that he was sober even at the end of the evening session. The second was that William Kelly was mistaken in recalling the amount of alcohol he and his brother drank that night, but again, James Kelly's sobriety does not tally with this explanation. The third was that after leaving the Oak Tree at about 10.45, reasonably sober and with a blood alcohol of about 150 milligrams, Kelly found some source of more alcohol, and drank enough of it to turn him into a roaring bull of a drunk. Examining this third suggestion, Benstead reckoned that if it were correct the final dose must have been taken at least three-quarters of an hour prior to his death – that is, in the period 10.45 to 11.15 p.m. This limited time, which would lead to the blood-alcohol level discovered in the corpse, would mean that the alcohol must have been in a concentrated form – that is, whisky, or some other spirit.

This theory is half supported by the half-bottle of whisky found on Kelly by the police. The missing half of that bottle would not have been enough to raise his blood alcohol level to 331 milligrams %, but the other half of the half-bottle could have been. So where did Kelly get that half-empty half-bottle? William said he definitely didn't have it on him when they parted company. Remember, though, that Kelly was lost sight of for a full hour and a quarter, so he had time enough to call at the back door of a friendly pub (where, without a penny in his pocket, he would have had to ask for the bottle on the slate) or knock up a friend and beg a drink. Or, as Benstead pointed out, all three explanations could be partially correct.

Benstead had delayed giving his view of the exact cause of death because he wanted to examine Kelly's heart. The microscope now revealed that the left coronary artery was three-quarters blocked and the right artery was half blocked. It didn't seem a complicated case – death was due to failure of the diseased heart, and the reason it occurred precisely when it did was through a combination of alcohol, emotion and exertion. He signed a death certificate to that effect, and in accordance with the usual practice the body was released to the family.

We must leave Benstead for a moment here and return to two unfortunate events that followed immediately after the death of Kelly that night and the post-mortem next day. The first of these concerned a policewoman attached to Huyton police station who was in fact a niece of Kelly. When she heard of her uncle's death she asked for, and received, permission to break the news initially to her parents as next of kin, rather than to Kelly's own mother, who was ill and alone at her home. She said that she was told by Sergeant Waddell that Kelly appeared to have suffered a heart attack, and she passed this information on to her parents. The family were later puzzled that the police could suggest a cause of death before a post-mortem had taken place. The fact that the police did not say at that time that the cause of death was a heart attack, but only that it appeared to be, seemed to escape everyone's attention.

The second event concerns Robert Kelly, a nephew

of the dead man, who said he was knocked up at home at about 1.45 p.m. on Thursday, June 21st, by two uniformed policemen and asked to identify from their description a man they told him had been found "lying in the road." Robert Kelly said, "That sounds like my Uncle James. Has he been in a fight?" One of the officers told him, "He's in a pretty serious condition." In fact, Kelly had already been dead in police custody for more than an hour when that conversation took place, and the suggestion that he had been found "lying in the road," with all the pacific connotation that phrase implies, was far from accurate. Why, the family wondered later, were the police less than frank on that occasion?

In the event no one should have been very much surprised when the Kelly family solicitors briefed Dr John Torry, a consultant pathologist in Wigan, to conduct a second post-mortem on their behalf. But Benstead *was* surprised, and he was also furious. The day that was chosen for Dr Torry's post-mortem coincided with a date in Benstead's diary on which he had to give evidence in a Crown Court case, which meant that he was unable to attend. This was an unusual circumstance, for in such cases one pathologist usually helps the other, and it was also unfortunate. In any event, Dr Torry's re-examination was bound to be incomplete because Benstead was in possession of Kelly's heart.

Something of Benstead's fury can be gauged from the fact that on Dr Torry's 17-page report of his examination of Kelly, Benstead wrote "Rubbish" nine times over nine different findings. But such internecine differences aside, Dr Torry's conclusions were markedly different from Benstead's. Dr Torry thought that "acute circulatory failure" was the main reason why Kelly died, but he listed two contributory factors: multiple injuries and alcoholic intoxication.

These factors, he held, rendered Kelly's death unnatural. For the vigilant Dr Torry had discovered something that appeared to be beyond contradiction – that Kelly's jaw was broken. The fracture had resulted from the blow recorded by Benstead in his injuries number six and seven. The fractured jaw, declared Dr Torry, would have given Kelly considerable pain ("Rubbish" chorused Benstead), and the blow which caused it was probably enough to bring about unconsciousness. There were other injuries that could have been significant. There was bruising in the right testicle which indicated either a blow to, or squeezing of, that testicle. (A policeman had admitted squeezing Kelly's testicles.) This squeezing could produce shock or sudden death, especially in a middle-aged man with severe heart disease. Kelly's injuries, declared Dr Torry, were "consistent with a severe beating." The only evidence of self-defence or assault he could find were bruises on two of Kelly's knuckles. Kelly would not have died in that short space of time, despite his heart disease and his high alcoholic content, if the incidents that took place on the night of his arrest had not happened.

Suddenly the case against the police looked menacing. Here is a man with a broken jaw who dies in police custody: rumours grew thick and fast in Huyton. Poor old Jim Kelly, who couldn't read or write and everyone knew was as drunk as a lord, had been beaten to death by the cops, and now they were all saying he'd had a heart attack and died naturally. The police pathologist had found 23 external marks on old Jim's body, but the family's pathologist found more than 40 – including a broken jaw. Poor old Jim – he never stood a chance in life and now he doesn't stand a chance in death ...

Benstead, aware that his back was to the wall, characteristically made a vigorous defence of his findings. The fractured jaw simply didn't matter, he argued, because it could not remotely have been held to be the cause of Kelly's death. Of course, it undoubtedly proved there was a hard blow to or on the chin. "But it is not the injury that matters, but the effect of the injury," he declared. "The hard blow to the jaw was a fact which was always appreciated and had the effects of it been serious they would have been apparent either in bruising or haemorrhage within the brain or inhalation of blood from the mouth into the lungs. Neither of these complications was present, albeit carefully and specifically looked for. Such fractures do not lead to any immediate significant disability. The victim may be unaware of the injury which may require only simple clamping; such injuries do not produce surgical shock. Indeed, the breaking of the jaw may even have cushioned any concussion effect on the brain. At Kelly's level of intoxication it is possible that the injury was not even noticed by Kelly himself."

But Dr Torry persisted. Two abrasions on Kelly's chest, he suggested, could have been caused by the same weapon, presumably a solid rod or bar about half an inch thick. This was pushing things a bit, because no weapon was found and the two marks could equally have been caused in many other ways – indeed, if a solid rod had been used on Kelly there would have been considerably more injury signs.

Benstead stuck by his view that the marks found on Kelly were trivial. Certainly Dr Torry listed more marks than Benstead, but that wasn't to say that Benstead didn't see them – he merely regarded them as inconsequential. As a result of these polarised views, a third examination of the body was made by Professor Alan Usher, who then wrote a detailed official report on how Kelly died. It was clear that even with the passage of time, when Professor Usher's report reached Benstead the pathologist was still seething. Professor Usher wrote, "Dr Torry's re-examination ... was long and extremely detailed ..." and Benstead wrote in the margin, "Not half! Five hours!" Dr Torry, said the Usher report, "also noted some bruising in the deep muscles of the back of the chest alongside the spine," for which Benstead's marginal note was "Unimportant!" The report drew attention to a small circular abrasion on Kelly's leg, the writer adding, "I cannot say exactly what caused this lesion," at the side of which Benstead wrote, "Neither can I!" – with what must have been something of a snort.

In fact, the official report agreed that most of those marks could have resulted from Kelly being punched or kicked or repeatedly knocked down by the police officers, and in view of the statements made by several of the witnesses that had to be considered a definite possibility. But, the report added with emphasis, there could also be several other possibilities. The marks could have been made in Kelly's coming into contact with the rough ground of the Barkbath Road waste land, with his contact with the police car, and with his lashing out at all and sundry in his drunken rage.

The independent report dealt with each of the 40-odd marks and summarised: "Even taken in total, they are certainly not injuries from which a normal adult would be expected to die. The usual brain contusions, intracranial haemorrhages, lacerations of the spleen, liver, kidneys and bladder which are present in persons who have been beaten or kicked to death were entirely absent in Kelly. Persons with fractured jaws usually walk into casualty departments and not infrequently, depending on the type and site of the fracture, require little in the way of treatment beyond simple pain-killing drugs." But the fractured jaw and the other minor injuries would have caused pain, and although at this time the drink Kelly had consumed would have dulled the pain, there could be little doubt that had he survived he would have had three or four very uncomfortable days, perhaps spent in bed.

It was pointed out too that late at night Kelly was an aggressive drunk in a tough neighbourhood where already episodes of violence involving unidentified people had been reported. How many times had he fallen down during the "missing period" – and what other difficulties had he got into? The police for their part didn't deny deliberately using violence; they justified it by saying that it was impossible to arrest him by any other means. Two of them were sufficiently badly injured to be forced to take a week off after the incident. The report concluded that "on the balance of probability" the primary cause of Kelly's death was "pre-existing natural heart disease."

"Fair enough," riposted Benstead. "But I am ultimately responsible to a Crown Court, and if I were to talk of balance of probability in court I should do so only once." The courtroom scene was never far from his mind. He once graphically described his initiation to cross-examination in court. He had just answered a difficult question using the words "one or two" when up leapt a defence barrister to ask, "Do you mean one or two, doctor? It may interest you to know that the difference is a hundred per cent."

The problem with the James Kelly case was that it got out of hand. His family and friends cared for him and were perfectly justified in requesting an inquiry into his death. What they were not to know was that others would see him as a convenient cause. Among the various political groups that tried to muscle in was the Workers' Revolutionary Party, with a Jimmy Kelly protest march. MPs rode hard on the issue of deaths in police custody (there were 245 cases in the previous decade, the 1970s), and Benstead's findings were twisted out of all recognition. He contemplated suing one national newspaper, and took counsel's opinion. The police did not help matters by retreating behind a wall of silence, but in the end they were vindicated. The independent report on Kelly's death also vindicated Benstead, and he let it rest there. Even the myth machine had failed to turn poor Jimmy Kelly into a martyr.

3

FORENSIC PSYCHIATRY

A shudder went round Broadmoor when it was learned that the most dangerous criminal lunatic in Britain had gone over the wall

A pathologist needs to be more than a diagnostician, a carver-up of bodies. He needs to have as well a fund of worldly wisdom, an accumulated insight into the dark and devious ways of the world. Take the case of the 16-year-old Lancashire student whose name we will withhold.

It had all the hallmarks of murder. A body, naked, bound and gagged, lying face down in the locked cubicle of a woman's toilet. The detectives who hurried to the scene drew in their breath and got ready to report a homicide. But this wasn't murder. It wasn't even suicide.

The body was discovered when a woman entered the tree-shrouded public toilets in Miller's Park, Preston, on a chilly Saturday morning in March. At the far end of the line of cubicles she saw two feet peeping out from under the gap between the bottom of the door and the floor. Frightened, she hurried off to call the police.

When the officers arrived they couldn't open the door, because the body was wedged against it. One of them climbed over the next cubicle, lowered himself into the end one and opened the door. The body lay face down with the head to the rear wall, and it was crammed between the side of the toilet bowl and the south wall. The clothing was stacked neatly on the far side of the toilet, together with the student's spectacles and belt.

A college scarf was bound around the toilet pipe and attached to the wrists behind the body. The ankles were also bound with a sock but the principal bindings surrounded the head, and they completely covered the young man's face.

These bindings were a pair of swimming trunks, rammed tightly over the head, a T shirt, sock and two handkerchiefs. One of the handkerchiefs was partly within the mouth, and the other had pushed back the tongue towards the throat.

While they were waiting for a doctor who had been summoned one of the police officers remarked, "There are a few bruises, but there doesn't seem any evidence of a struggle." The bruises, he thought, might have been caused by the young man himself in his death throes.

The doctor made notes, observing that some of the young man's pubic hair had been shaved. Then he wrote, "I have found no direct evidence from my examination of the scene in Miller's Park to indicate that any other person was involved in the death of this student."

As the doctor left the scene Benstead arrived. He strolled jauntily into the ladies' toilet, now roped off by the police, and studied the body, spread out on a plastic sheet on the floor alongside the cubicles. Rigor mortis was advanced and the body (which had lain on the lavatory floor since the previous afternoon) was very cold. He made a preliminary examination, then ordered the body to be sent to Royal Preston Hospital for a post-mortem.

In the hospital's morgue Benstead found nothing unusual about the youngster's internal organs – liver, lungs, spinal cord, heart were normal. So, too, he wrote, was the brain. But he knew when he wrote this that he was thinking only as a physician. If he could have seen inside that brain, read its last thoughts, he would have known a great deal more about the student's death.

As it was, he could only write, "In my opinion death resulted from 1, asphyxia and 2, hypothermia." Then he added significantly, "It is further my opinion that the circumstances of this death were characteristic of a well known abnormal behaviour pattern and that there is no evidence or indication that any other person was involved."

The student was the victim of the phenomenon of self-inflicted asphyxia for sexual gratification. This form of death is not uncommon, and results when adolescent boys – and, much more rarely, adult men – die from strangulation or hanging after tying themselves up and indulging in various masochistic practices. There is of course no intention to commit suicide – the awareness of sexual pleasure is apparently heightened by the restriction of oxygen to the brain. But the pleasure-seeker is in grave danger, for what sometimes follows is a condition called inhibition of the vagal nerve – the nerve which supplies the heart, lungs and viscera, and it is this condition which prevents the victim from freeing himself. He loses consciousness rapidly and death occurs from asphyxia. In cases of suspected sexually motivated asphyxia the forensic scientist looks for supportive evidence, such as signs of masturbation and the presence of pornographic literature or women's clothing near the body.

Two murder cases from John Benstead's casebook reflect the kind of society we created in the late years of the twentieth century. The first contains elements still very much in discussion today – how much freedom if any are we to give to mentally ill criminals? Probably the first big clamorous cry of alarm on this subject came from a frightened public when the child-killer John Straffen, 22, escaped from Broadmoor Hospital.

A shudder went round that institution on Tuesday, April 29th, 1952, when it was learned that Straffen, then undoubtedly the most dangerous man in Broadmoor – which made him the most dangerous criminal lunatic in Britain – had gone over the wall to freedom. He had been incarcerated for killing two little girls after the trial judge, referring to the prisoner's mental age, told the jury, "You might as well try a babe in arms." Everyone in Broadmoor knew that if Straffen escaped the first thing he would do would be to kill again.

And that is exactly what he did that April afternoon. He found a five-year-old girl playing on her new bicycle, took her to a wood, and strangled her under an oak tree with his bare hands. Medical evidence suggested that it took between 15 to 30 seconds for the child to die after pressure had been applied to her throat. There was no sexual interference; the murder was a carbon copy of the other two for which Straffen had been sentenced. Forty minutes later he was recaptured. He told police officers that he had escaped to prove that he could be out without killing children. He was taken back to the institution and locked in his cell for the night. The pathetic body of the little girl was not discovered until the next day.

Straffen told police that he didn't feel sorry about killing his latest victim – "I had no feeling about it." He never made any secret of his motivation for all three killings, which was his hatred of the police, who were always out to get him.

Straffen's case belonged to the realms of forensic psychiatry, the newest of the forensic disciplines, particularly in its field of attempting to understand the motivations to violence. He was a mental defective – and mental defect is defined by law as a condition of arrested development of mind occurring before the age of 18. It is virtually always congenital, but Parliament decided on a definition which would include arrested development starting in childhood. It is usually regarded as synonymous with intellectual defect – that is, an inability to learn. Straffen was regarded as having a "low-grade feeble mind" with a mental age of nine, at the lower end of the scale of the class of defectives who are defined as "needing care and supervision for the sake of themselves and others." An adult with a mental age of nine is, of course, a very different proposition from a child of nine. He has had a great deal more experience, and he is usually emotionally – especially sexually – very much more developed.

From the medico-legal angle, Straffen's case brought out a peculiar anomaly. Committal to an institution because of mental deficiency was an alternative to a prison sentence, on the obvious ground that the prisoner was not considered to be properly responsible for his acts. But in 1951 the law allowed no such alternative to a capital offence. Therefore the only medical disposal possible was committal to Broadmoor on grounds of insanity. In a court of law this meant proving he was insane under the M'Naghten Rules, which lay down that if a murderer knows what he is doing is wrong at the time he kills, then he is not insane.

The arguments between the doctors and the lawyers over Straffen then turned on the interpretation of the meaning of a "disease of the mind." Was the defect of reason, from which Straffen clearly suffered to be attributed to a disease of the mind? Dr. J. C. Matheson, medical officer at Brixton Prison, held, in company with many other doctors, that there was no disease of the mind.

That seemed to many people at the time to be open to challenge. Straffen was clearly guilty under the M'Naghten Rules, for in killing the little girls he knew what he did, and he knew that his acts were wrong – his motive for it was to annoy the police. So it was fair to ask, especially when he was sentenced to be hanged for the third murder, can it really be contended that murdering children in order to annoy the police is consistent with true sanity? Superficially he appeared a dreadful murderer. Yet looked at with a sense of detachment, the very degree of callousness was evidence of a deranged mind.

However, the authorities who regarded his behaviour simply in terms of moral obliquity appeared to win the day against Straffen. Their outraged impotence was first revealed when he appeared in court after his escape with a large bruise on the side of his face. No one asked how it happened – yet even in Victorian times pointed questions were asked about the beating-up of mental defectives.

When Straffen was brought to trial for the murder of the first two little girls he was considered unfit to plead and sent to Broadmoor. At his second trial he was not found "guilty but insane," as he should have been if there was any consistency in his case, but "guilty" and sentenced to death. Hours before he was due to be executed he was reprieved, and in due course sent back to Broadmoor, this time after being certified as a mental defective in jail. Straffen indeed was always a mental defective, and as soon as he revealed himself to be a dangerous one, deserved to be treated as such. What went on after his escape and recapture was a unique series of happenings in English law, which sadly brought little credit to that law.

The case of John Straffen must have crossed the mind of Dr. Benstead when he stared down at the body of Janice McKinley, lying naked in a small wood in front of Rainhill Hospital, a place where the mentally ill are treated.

Janice, slightly built, with long dark hair, was 22. She had gone into the hospital as a voluntary patient, and now she was lying dead in the hospital grounds from the effects of a horrendous knife wound. A gash three inches wide across her throat penetrated to the right side of her spine, almost severing her head from her body. In addition, a second gash had cut through her abdomen to the small intestine. Other small cuts and abrasions were visible on her body.

Death, Benstead quickly decided, was due to haemorrhage and shock caused by the terrible throat wound. How long she had taken to die was an imponderable – "it is difficult to assess how much blood has soaked into the ground," he wrote in his notes.

He noticed a pool of blood, though, a few inches to one side of the body. Did this mean that the body had been moved? "It is easier to turn a body in rigor mortis," he wrote at the scene of the crime. "Did the killer come back and inflict some more cuts on her after she was dead?" There certainly were more cuts besides the one that caused her death.

Janice had not been raped or sexually assaulted – and this, together with the evidence that her murderer killed her savagely, then perhaps returned to stab her again – pointed to a maniac.

Scattered through the wood were the remnants of her clothing. Where her body lay among the dead leaves and bracken she was completely naked. This would not have been voluntary in the bitterly cold last days of January.

Benstead raised his eyes to survey the immediate vicinity. A wide, rutted path led out of the wood towards a distant building – Rainhill Hospital, a place of refuge and treatment for the mentally ill.

Janice had last been seen by hospital staff on the morning of the previous day, Sunday. At lights-out on Sunday evening she was reported missing and the hue and cry was raised. She was found dead in the wood early the next day. The trail of forensic evidence led police to Samuel Vincent Packer, aged 43, who had been recently released from "a top-security mental unit" called Scott Clinic, in the grounds of the hospital.

Packer's trial was to raise questions which would not go away. Under pressure from Janice's parents and their legal advisors an inquiry was set up by the Mersey Regional Health Authority under the chairmanship of Bruce Martin QC. It did not publish its findings until October, 1986 – twenty months after the murder – but it was scathing in the width and breadth of its attack on officials and officialdom, blaming a series of errors by an unnamed forensic psychiatrist, the Home Office, senior managers at the secure unit where Packer was kept, and the district health authority.

But the public never knew the full details of the mistakes that led to Packer being allowed to wander freely on parole from Scott Clinic in the hospital grounds. For the investigators' report was kept secret. Only their recommendations were published. And they said that no one should be disciplined in the wake of the tragic killing – provided tough new rules were introduced. These would be based on the inquiry's own proposals, which it was claimed would make the people of Rainhill safe from psychopaths in the secure Scott Clinic.

"We have no doubt that if our recommendations are

implemented in full the risk of another case having such a tragic end as that of Packer should be very substantially reduced," the report said. "This should ensure that those living nearby to such a clinic should be at least as safe – if not safer – than in the community at large."

The investigators made 40 recommendations, including a complete revision of all operational policies of the Scott Clinic, the Home Office to be told if a patient is involved in a serious incident, psychopaths to be offered treatment only after very careful assessment, regular liaison between the clinic and the police, and the Home Office to make more information on patients available. A spokesman for the regional health authority, which set up the inquiry and whose district health authority was one of the institutions blamed for Janice's death, then said, "We will do everything humanly possible to ensure that another tragedy does not happen again."

Not surprisingly, not everyone was placated by phrases like "the risk...should be very substantially reduced" and "We will do everything possible to ensure that another tragedy does not happen again," because such phrases do not imply that the system will in future be foolproof, and taken together with the "no one's to blame" attitude they smacked of a big bureaucratic cover-up. And cover-up was the phrase used when the murder was raised in Parliament.

A few days after the inquiry's recommendations were made public, Frank Field, M.P. for Birkenhead, asked the then Health Minister, Douglas Hogg, why the report shouldn't be published in its entirety. But the minister wouldn't have it. He replied, "The question of publication is a matter for the Mersey Regional Health Authority."

Janice McKinley's father was subsequently allowed to see a copy of the report. The rest of the nation wasn't so lucky. Not even Dr John Benstead saw it. We still don't know what went on at the Scott Clinic, and we are not going to be told. But reviewing all the silky-smooth platitudes that came out of the inquiry into the horrific murder of Janice, people will ask, as Mr. McKinley asked, "Will someone else's daughter be murdered by a maniac who should never have been released upon society?" It is of course a rhetorical question.

4

PUTTING THE BODY TOGETHER AGAIN

As the holidaymaker gazed at the spectacular scene her gaze narrowed. On a rock below was a broken parcel—and from it protruded a human leg

While it is comparatively easy to extinguish life in the human body, the body itself remains a difficult object to destroy. Many infamous murderers have tried it and failed, because almost always something is left for the forensic scientst to work on. But these are the murderers we know about. How many, one wonders, got away with it – leaving bits of their victim's corpse scattered across the land?

The dismembered, disarticulated, mutilated mortal remains of killers' victims are the working models for forensic scientists. These experts have to be clinical, unemotional, strong-stomached and meticulously observant about their work in a way perhaps best summed up by the pathologist Sir Bernard Spilsbury's famous remark before dissecting a corpse in his laboratory, "Shut the window. I like to be able to smell the smells that tell me something."

The most difficult task confronting forensic scientists is the putting together of a body which has been cut up by the killer and scattered around in a variety of different places. If the bones only are available the problems increase, for it is not always easy to say whether certain bones belong to the same skeleton or not. If the soft parts are attached to them, that makes things slightly easier. The first objective on discovery is to make sure that the remains are human. In one recorded case, for example, when a tin box found in a ditch was prised open it was seen to contain a windpipe ten inches long attached to lungs. The tongue and heart had been cut off. A doctor was called to examine the remains and decided that they came from a child. A forensic scientist soon put him right – the adult human windpipe measures at most five inches. The remains were probably from a calf.

In cases where only muscle or viscera are found, forensic scientists use a test on the protein matter called the precipitin test, by which they can determine whether the matter is human or otherwise. John George Haigh, the Crawley acid bath murderer, thought he could get rid of his victims' bodies completely by dropping them into a vat of strong commercial sulphuric acid and then pouring the residue over the yard where he was working. He nearly succeeded, for interaction of the water in body tissue and the commercial acid he was using created a great deal of heat, reducing the bodies to sludge. But Professor Keith Simpson had the yard dug up and removed the top three inches of a soil over an area of nearly 50 yards. This was packed up and sent to his laboratory. He sifted out 457 pounds of greasy sludge, and isolated 28 pounds of yellow fat from it – all that remained of Haigh's victims. In one tray of fat Simpson found a set of dentures, in another he found three gallstones. In one of the gallstones there was sufficient protein matter to give a positive human precipitin test. One of Haigh's possible victims, Mrs. Olive Durand-Deacon, was known to suffer from gallstones, and the dentures were soon identified as hers by her dentist. So the police were already on their way to discovering that at least one body had been destroyed in the vat of acid, and who the victim was.

Having discovered that the remains are human, the forensic scientist must decide whether they belong to one body or more. This isn't as easy as it sounds, because different stages of putrefaction can occur according to the locality where a part was found, and even where some of the parts are found together the limbs are usually less putrefied than the trunk of the same body.

Putrefaction itself has given rise to many studies, as a result of which forensic scientists know that dead bodies pass through certain stages of disintegration. Hypostasis, or lividity, starts about four hours after death, and is caused by the sinking, through gravity, of the red corpuscles in the blood to the lowest part of the body. If the body is found in a standing position, for instance, hypostasis is found in the legs and feet; if, as is more general, it is lying on its back, hypostasis would be found in the back. Hypostasis is revealed by a general discoloration, or lividness, of the skin. After about five hours rigor mortis sets in, descending from the head downwards through the body over a period of about 18 hours, and leaving the body in the same order over the next 18 hours. Putrefaction begins after two days with staining and distending of the body. After three weeks vesicles and organs start to burst. Adipocere, a kind of hard, white, suety substance unpleasant to the touch, is formed from the body fats, and, if the conditions are damp is visible after four months, first on the face and head; it spreads to the trunk after six months. It should be stressed that the forensic pathologist would know these timings are approximate, and in order to arrive at his conclusions would make certain amendments to the rules depending on temperature, weather conditions (if the body is found outside), whether the corpse was that of a young person or an old one, whether it was diseased at death or in good health, and other factors.

Curiously, in the nineteenth century when parts of a human corpse were discovered the cause was often set down as being the work of anatomical preparations by a medical student. There must have been some killers who dismembered their victims and got away with it because for lack of scientific knowledge or any evidence to the contrary the police decided that the bits of body were no more than the material used by some budding doctor to further his knowledge. And of course if a doctor himself decided to turn killer, he was always able to claim that any bits of human body found on his premises were there for research purposes. One such case in the nineteenth century involved a certain Professor Webster, and it has become a landmark in modern forensic detection.

On Friday, November 23rd, 1849, a doctor named Parkman went to Professor Webster's laboratory in Boston, and was never seen again. Detectives who went to the laboratory a week later found hidden in a vault two hip bones, a right thigh, and a lower left leg. In a furnace they found portions of bones, bits of vertebrae, and artificial teeth. In a tea chest they found the entire trunk of a human body which had apparently been immersed in formaldehyde. When all these parts were placed together they were seen to belong to one body. The body had not undergone any dissection for anatomical purposes, and the parts had been cut and hacked about by someone with only limited knowledge of the human body. It was calculated that the portions belonged to a man between fifty and sixty years old, and measurements of the vertebrae suggested that he would be a fraction under five feet eleven inches. Dr. Parkman in fact was sixty years old and stood five feet eleven inches.

Professor Webster was arrested and, clearly much alarmed by all these new-fangled deductions, protested that the findings were based entirely on circumstantial evidence, that the identity of the remains had not been established satisfactorily, and no cause of death was proved. The jury were unconvinced by his protests and found him guilty, and he was executed. It is interesting to note from this case that Dr. Parkman's head, feet and hands – the parts which are generally most needed to identify a victim – were missing and never found, and yet identity was still established.

Joining the parts exactly together – the jigsaw process of forensic science in dismembering cases – is vital to the case for the prosecution. Even before the Boston case of Professor Webster this fact was being recognised by English jurists. In 1837 a man named James Greenacre murdered a woman, sawed off her head and her limbs from the trunk and scattered the parts across London. The limbs were not found until six weeks after the discovery of the trunk, presenting a problem which must have taxed the limited knowledge of doctors in the first part of the nineteenth century. Even so, they examined the trunk carefully and noticed that the fifth cervical vertebra had been almost sawn through, leaving only about a tenth of an inch of that bone. When they looked at the head they saw that the fifth cervical vertebra had also been partly sawn through, leaving nine-tenths in situ. The two parts fitted exactly, even to the continuation of a superficial cut on the skin.

The thigh bones had been sawn through half-way, then broken off. When the trunk was put alongside the legs the cut surfaces and the jagged, broken-off surfaces exactly fitted. All this forensic work was confirmed by the discovery that the woman did not have a uterus – which was known to be the case with the woman whom Greenacre was suspected of killing. Greenacre, no doubt bewildered by all his cutting-up work coming to nothing, was hanged.

A hundred years later in the celebrated case known as the Brighton trunk murder the head and later the body of a woman were found in different and distant places. A pathologist noted that there were four cervical vertebrae attached to the body and three to the head. He noted too that the divided vessels and cartilaginous rings of the windpipe fitted together exactly. When the pieces were put together the woman was identified.

When a dismembered body that has clearly lain unnoticed for some time is found the pieces are then generally treated for maggot-infestation and left to soak in a formalin solution.

Some murderers who dismember their victims boil or burn or treat the parts with chemicals to hasten decomposition, so a forensic scientist must watch out for any such tell-tale signs. If vital organs have been found, he must also be on the look-out for any indications of injury that might have caused death, or any injuries that might have been inflicted after death.

Some murderers who dismember will go to inordinate lengths to render their victim unrecognisable. Often, though, they make some mistake, either through panic or from inexpertise, that leads to their arrest. But sometimes they do such an expert job they get clean away with it. Such a one was the killer who stopped on Waterloo Bridge in October, 1857, and lowered a dismembered corpse in a bag over the side, intending it to float away in the river. But something went wrong, alhough the killer walked off evidently satisfied with his night's work. He must have been unaware that the bag of human remains was stuck in one of the bridge's buttresses, where it was found next day.

There were 23 human parts in the bag, chiefly of bones with flesh attached to them, and they had been sawn into very small pieces. The total weight of the parts was only 18 pounds – about one-eighth of the average weight of an adult body at that time. The flesh had been roughly cut from the bones. The trunk, including part of the chest and spine, had been cut into eight pieces, the upper limbs had been cut or sawn into six, and the lower limbs into nine pieces. The head and fourteen out of 24 vertebrae were missing, as well as the hands and feet and some parts of the chest. The killer was obviously determined to leave absolutely no evidence that would lead to the identity of his victim – evidence that might thereafter lead to his own identity as well.

The first thing that was obvious was that the body belonged to a male, since a portion of the sex organs, which were severely mutilated, was still attached to the pelvis. The bones had been sawn through near the joints, evidently with great trouble, with a fine bone-saw, such as then used by bone-boilers. They had been probably cut and sawn before the rigidity of death had completely ceased – say about 18 hours. On the chest there was a stab which looked as if it might have penetrated the heart; this wound had been inflicted while the man was still alive. The spinal cord had been violently torn out of the vertebral canal. Portions of the muscle, skin and ligaments were brown and sodden, and gave the impression of having been boiled in water and soaked in a solution of salt. The portions of skin remaining were covered thickly with dark hairs. The bones were fully developed, so by measuring them and adding approximations for the missing parts the pathologist was able to deduce that this adult man was 5 feet 9 inches tall. He was also able to say that the man had been dead for three or four weeks, and that he was dark and hairy.

Besides the human remains found in the bag suspended from the bridge there were some fragments of clothing indicating several stab wounds, and indicating as well that the man was a foreigner. With only this information to go on, the police started inquiries. They discovered that three weeks previously a Swedish sailor had disappeared from his ship moored in the river. And there the trail ended. Despite the mistake he made on Waterloo Bridge, the killer got away with it. Who he was, and why the sailor – if it was him – was set upon and stabbed to death, was never discovered.

The forensic scientists' classic case of dismemberment went into the text-books in the 1930s, when the remains of two bodies were discovered by a holiday visitor to Scotland. Susan Johnson had set off from her hotel after lunch, determined to make the most of her last two days' holiday. She strode down the A6 road linking Edinburgh and Carlisle towards the Gardenholme Linn valley, just outside Moffat in the border country. The autumn light coloured the surrounding hills and gave the Scottish landscape that special glow that stays long afterwards in the mind's eye.

Miss Johnson paused on a bridge and gazed down at the spectacular Gardenholme ravine. Then her gaze narrowed. Quite visible on a rock below was a broken parcel. And from it protruded a human leg. She took one more look, screamed, and ran back to her hotel to fetch her brother. He climbed down over the rocks into the ravine and confirmed what she had seen.

Quickly summoned, the police found several more parcels of human remains – and down the Linn river in the next few days they were to find a dozen more. All the parcels appeared to have been tossed into the Linn, and all were suddenly revealed because the river, a rain-swollen torrent a few days earlier, was now just a trickle.

The police called in two local doctors for an outline report, together with Dr. Alexander Mearns, of the

Institute of Hygiene at the University of Glasgow, who wrote a report on the maggot-infestation of the body parts. Three types of maggots are usually found on decaying flesh. The common bluebottle and the common greenbottle prefer to lay their eggs in groups of about 150, to a maximum of 2,000 eggs, on fresh rather than putrefied flesh. The eggs hatch usually within a day, then another day passes, the first skin is shed and another larva appears. Still another larva appears after another three days, and yet another appears seven days later – and each new larva is larger than its predecessor. The final larva feeds for another five days, then leaves the body, buries itself in the ground and pupates, after which the new fly is born, usually in the spring. The house-fly maggot is involved in a similar cycle, although there are essential differences in times. It can be seen from this that once the larvae in decaying flesh are identified the forensic scientist has a vital time-of-death clue which he can deduce from the development stage of the larvae.

On October 1st, 1935, two days after the discovery of the first human parcel in the Linn river, two forensic scientists, Professor John Glaister and Dr. Millar, arrived from Edinburgh to make a detailed examination. They washed the remains in a bath, treated them with ether to destroy the maggots which heavily infested them, and placed them in a weak solution of formalin in locked tanks, where they remained for three days. The two experts then had the remains removed to the laboratory of the forensic scientist Sir Sydney Smith, whose name was to become famously linked with the case. Carefully they put together the pieces and made two bodies of them – one female and the other male – which they called Body No. 1 and Body No. 2.

In Body No. 1 the head had been severed from the trunk immediately below the chin. Since it was deduced that the killer was using only a knife, it was immediately clear that he knew exactly how to go about his grisly work. The head had been severely mutilated by removal of skin and underlying tissues; the nose and both ears had been cut off, and both eyes removed, the lips had been almost entirely cut away, the two upper central incisor teeth had been drawn and the hair had been roughly shaved.

In Body No. 2 the head had been severed from the trunk at a level a little lower than in the case of Body No. 1. The mutilation of the head was much more extensive. Not only the nose, both ears, and both eyes but also nearly the whole of the skin of the head and face had been removed. Both lips had been completely removed, and nearly all the teeth had been drawn. The swollen tongue protruded between the jaws, and the tip had been cut off.

The trunk had been divided into two portions. As was the case with Body No. 1, the arms had been disarticulated at the shoulder joints. The bottom half of the trunk, including the whole of the pelvis and most of its organs, had been cut out. As also was the case with Body No. 1, the thighs had been disarticulated at the hip joints, and most of the skin and soft tissues, including the external genital organs, had been removed from the pelvis.

The two experts made some other remarkable deductions. Both victims had been asphyxiated. In both cases great care had been take to remove all identification marks. And they had both been dismembered with such precision that their killer must have been someone with medical knowledge and skill.

But he had left some vital clues. Some parts of the body were wrapped in a yellow jumper, and some in a child's romper suit. Other parts were wrapped in a copy of the *Sunday Graphic*, dated only four days earlier, September 15th, 1935, and that particular issue was a special limited edition for the Morecambe Bay carnival, delivered only in Morecambe and Lancaster. These two towns were 125 miles from the discovery of the grisly remains.

Thus it was reasonable for the police to assume that this killer with medical knowledge had murdered the two people in Lancashire, then driven up the A6 as far as he thought was necessary, looking for a river in which to dump the dismembered pieces. The problem, though, was that both bodies were beyond all identification.

At Lancaster police station, news of the Moffat discovery struck a chord. Not two people but just one woman had been reported missing there. She was Mary Jane Rogerson, 21, who had vanished in mid-September. She was nanny to the children of Dr. Buck Ruxton, a Parsee Indian G.P. practising in Dalton Square, Lancaster. Dr. Ruxton had told Mary's worried parents that she had left his employ because she was pregnant. They thought that so out of character for their daughter that they didn't believe him.

It was short work for Mary's parents to identify the yellow jumper found in the parcels as their daughter's. The were also able to say that the child's romper suit had belonged to the Ruxtons' youngest child. But whose was the other body?

Just at the point where Lancaster police decided to go and have word with Dr. Ruxton, he went to see them.

"My wife Isabella has disappeared," he said. "She went in my car to see the Blackpool illuminations on Saturday, September 14th. I found the car abandoned next day, Sunday. Please help me."

It wasn't necessary to probe too deeply into the Ruxtons' family life to discover they were a quarrelsome couple. Indeed, the police may well have remembered the troublesome doctor's previous calls on their time. A year earlier Ruxton called at the police station after his wife had made a complaint against him, flew into a violent temper, accused his wife of being unfaithful, and added, "I would be justified in murdering her." Later he told the police, "My wife has been unfaithful and I will kill her if it continues."

On a third occasion, only six months before the discovery of the human remains, he told a police officer, "I feel like murdering two people in Dalton Square. My wife is going out to meet another man."

The Ruxton family, it seemed, fairly rocked with violence. Once, when Mrs. Ruxton left the house taking all her clothes Ruxton told a maid, "She won't come back alive. I will bring her back to the mortuary." Another maid told the police that she had seen the doctor holding his wife down on their bed with his hands around her throat. He ran from the room calling his wife "a dirty prostitute."

The nub of Ruxton's jealousy was his conviction that his wife was having an affair with a local town hall solicitor, Robert Edmundson, a man described as "of irreproachable character." Early in September 1935 Mrs. Ruxton went to Edinburgh with a party of people which included Mr. Edmundson. Unbeknown to them, Ruxton followed in his car, with brown paper pasted on the windscreen to avoid recognition. The party travelled over the bridge beneath which the remains of the two bodies were later found. It was an innocent expedition, but Ruxton returned with the idea that his wife had stayed the night with Mr. Edmundson.

So if Mrs. Isabella Ruxton had suffered the same fate as her maid, and Ruxton was the killer, it would be safe to assume that jealousy was the motive. Then more servants made statements which seemed to point to Ruxton being involved in some way and for whatever reason in the death of Mary Rogerson. Elizabeth Curwen and Agnes Oxley both said they were given the weekend of September 14th - 15th off by Dr. Ruxton. Another servant said that on Sunday, September 15th, Dr. Ruxton had his hand bandaged, explaining that he had jammed it in a door.

That explanation might have been accepted had it not been for the fact that for the rest of that Sunday, Ruxton told a series of different stories to different people about his activities. He told a neighbour who agreed to look after his three children that day that he had cut his hand opening a tin of fruit. Then he drove to the house of a patient, Mrs. Mary Hampshire. "Would you help me?" he asked. "Mary Robertson has gone on holiday and my wife is staying in Blackpool. I've cut my hand and I can't get the house ready for the decorators."

Mrs. Hampshire went back with him and was stunned by the state of the house. There was no carpet on the stairs and landing and there was straw right up to the top floor. She cleaned the bath, which was filthy. In the backyard she saw the stairs and landing carpets, which were heavily bloodstained. There were also two towels and a shirt, all bloodstained, and half burned.

Later that day the doctor gave Mrs. Hampshire's husband a bloodstained blue suit. Next morning he called again on the Hampshires. They thought he looked "very ill," and were somewhat astonished when he asked if he could have back the suit so that he could get it cleaned. Mr. Hampshire told him that was unnecessary, that he had already been kind enough, and he would have it cleaned at his own expense. Nonetheless, Ruxton asked for the suit and some scissors, and carefully cut out the maker's name from the jacket before giving it back to Mr. Hampshire.

As all these statements built up in the Ruxton file at Lancaster police station, Dr. Ruxton was still free, still continuing with his practice. What the police wanted positively to establish above all else was the identity of the second victim, and the whereabouts of Mrs. Isabella Ruxton.

In one brief, enlightening moment all the pieces of the jig-saw suddenly came together. At the Moffat mortuary Professor Glaister suddenly realised that the bodies were not those of a man and a woman but of two women. As the murderer cut up the bodies he had tried to destroy all evidence of sex. But he had made some oversights. Among the seventy pieces of flesh and fat he left three female breasts and portions of sex organs which revealed that two women were involved.

The killer's blunders, Sir Sydney Smith decided, were, despite the detailed work of dismemberment, undertstandable, because of the time it must have taken to cut up and mutilate the two bodies. At the murder trial Sydney Smith agreed with Professor Glaister's estimate that the dismemberment and disarticulation of Body No. 2 would have taken about five hours; later, in his autobiography, Sydney Smith estimated that the dismemberment, disarticulation and mutilation of both bodies would have taken a total of eight hours. He was to recall later, when the Parsee doctor had been established as the murderer, "One can well imagine Ruxton's state of mind with that mass of flesh and bones in his bathroom. It looked sufficiently formidable to me when I saw it first in my laboratory. The worry it must have induced was sufficient reason for his overlooking so many details and making so many blunders."

How had the two experts arrived at the time for cutting up Body No. 2? Sydney Smith said that he and Professor Glaister had gone over the various operations part by part and reckoned out the time they would themselves probably take to do the same amount of stripping and disarticulation. The general evidence was eventually to show that Ruxton must have started cutting up the bodies at soon after midnight on the Sunday, and the time available to him to finish the job would have run out at about 4 p.m. – hence he had more than enough of the time estimated by the two forensic pathologists.

Working with Professor John Brash, Professor Glaister painstakingly put together the two bodies. Body No. 1, the two experts concluded, was about 4 ft. 11 ins. tall and aged between 18 and 25. Mary Rogerson was in fact 5 ft. tall and 21 years old.

Body No. 2, which was the one first thought to be male, was about 5ft. 3 ins. and aged between 35 and 45. Isabella Ruxton was 5ft. 5 ins. and 34 years old.

The bodies had been drained of their blood. They had also been indiscriminately mutilated and the reason could only be arrived at by examining the known facts about the physical condition of the two women. In Body No. 1 the eyes and the upper forearm skin had been removed. Mary Rogerson had a squint in one eye, and a distinctive birthmark on her upper forearm. In Body No. 2 the fingernails, soft leg tissue and teeth had been removed, tissue had been excised from part of the right thumb, and the left foot was badly mutilated. Isabella Ruxton had noticeably square fingernails, shapeless legs, prominent teeth and a scar on her right thumb; she also had a bunion and toes bent in a recognisable way. The killer had incidentally overlooked the fact that a bunion can leave an identifiable bone deformity, as had happened in the case of Body No. 2. He had also overlooked the fact that by deliberately destroying important identification features in each of the two bodies he was actually drawing attention to the points he was trying to conceal.

The initial problem of gender identity came about because it took time to recognise three of the separate soft parts as female breasts. Two of them seemed to form a pair and some attempt, unconvincing in its result, was made to fit them together from the appearance of their skin edges and attach them to the trunk of Body No. 2. From one of the breasts the nipple and surrounding areolar area had been excised. The third breast was not so easily recognised. It was covered with skin in which there was a gaping, irregular wound, about four inches long, where the nipple had apparently been cut out.

The police now had a case – some might think an overwhelming one. Ruxton, it was assumed, had got into another violent row with his wife on the Saturday night. Bruises on the remains showed that he had beaten her up, then killed her by asphyxiating her. But why did Mary Rogerson have to die? The only assumption is that she saw what was happening to her mistress, and Ruxton in his murderous frenzy decided to silence her. She had blows to the head that fractured her skull, but she had been killed by some other means.

Ruxton then opened the bodies and drained them of their blood into the bath, leaving it in the state seen by Mrs. Hampshire. Having parcelled them up, he locked them in two rooms at the top of the house before taking them up the A6 to Moffat – a route with which, ironically, he would have been familiar as a result of his shadowing his wife on her Edinburgh night out.

On the day before his arrest he was busying himself around his patients in Lancaster trying to establish alibis, many of which conflicted with each other. He asked a decorator who he had called to his home to say if he were asked that he had been booked some weeks earlier. The decorator had in fact been booked earlier – but to decorate a different room.

A reporter who interviewed Ruxton at his home said, "He paced up and down the library floor, ran trembling fingers through tousled hair, and occasionally thumped his forehead with the palm of his hand. Now and again he stopped, swung round, and almost screamed, 'I did not kill my Belle; I tell you she has gone away, she will come back.'

"Then he sobbed, 'Tell everyone I am not guilty. Tell them I loved my Belle too much to harm her.'"

Ruxton showed the police two typewritten sheets headed "My movements." The entry dated Sunday, September 15th – the day after the murder – read,

"Mrs. R suggested going for a day's trip. I agreed. Asked me to get up and go for the car. I went to the garage, took the car out... It was a little after seven. I began getting ready slowly. Isabella and Mary were both upstairs when I was in the bathroom. Isabella then asked if I mind her going to Edinburgh that day instead of the day after. I said jokingly, 'Are you sure you know what to do? All right, please yourself, but you will have to go without my car.' She said, 'I am taking Mary with me.' I felt rather glad at that because I said to myself that if she goes with Mary she is sure to come back, because Mrs. R has been hinting that one day she will go away for good. It was about half-past nine when they left. She shouted, 'There is a cup of tea on the hall table for you.'"

He described too how he fetched a tin of peaches, "Brought it up to the bedroom and in attempting to open it mashed my right-hand fingers. Detailed account of this already with the police."

The police must have thought that Ruxton was working overtime to explain himself, remembering every phrase in his conversation with his wife, his every reaction to something he was told. They began checking his past. He was born Bukhtyark Rustomji Ratanji Hakim in Bombay, the son of a wealthy Indian doctor and a French mother. He began his studies at London University, but problems with his spoken English decided him to complete his medical course at Bombay Medical College.

In Bombay he married a Parsee Indian woman and when he returned to England as an Indian Army doctor he left his Indian wife behind. Isabella, manageress of a cafe, was in fact his common-law wife. She was also legally married, to a Dutchman with whom she lived for only a few months.

Captain Hakim, as Ruxton was then called, decided to buy a general practice in Lancaster, where his three children were born to Isabella. But Isabella never knew about the Indian marriage of her "Bommie," as she called him, and Ruxton was always fearful that she would find out about it. Within a few years he was earning £3,000 a year, an excellent salary in the early Thirties, but he handled money badly, and for a time Isabella worked as manageress of a Woolworth's cafeteria in Edinburgh.

The doctor changed his name by deed poll to Buck Ruxton, but his patients, for whom an Indian doctor was much more of a rarity then than is the case today, called him "The Rajah." Perhaps because his generosity to his patients – these were the days when everyone had to pay the doctor – was legendary in his practice he found himself increasingly in debt and in the hands of moneylenders.

Ruxton was evidently a very popular doctor, but hopelessly unable to control his emotions. His violent rages would frequently culminate in his bursting into tears. His jealousy was so overwhelming that he was said to have forced Isabella to run barefoot up and down stairs 50 times because she had danced with another man at a local event.

This was the man who was brought to trial at Manchester Assizes in March, 1936. He was charged only with the murder of Isabella Ruxton. In the witness-box he gave a concise summary of his stormy relations with his wife: "We were the sort of people who could not live with each other or without each other." Every time a quarrel arose with his wife, he said, "I paid dearly for it." After the quarrels their relations were "more than intimate", and his wife would come to him smiling and say, "Why did we kick up a row?"

Asked about a bruise on Mrs. Ruxton's arm, Ruxton burst into tears and said, "Must I answer it? I will if you want me to." He added, "I saw my Isabella with a photograph of a man. I said, 'Isabella, what are you hiding? I did not attack her, but when I snatched it I may have caused the bruise."

The blood on the stair carpet, he thought, must have come from his cut hand. The carpets were pulled up and the decorator arrived next day. Explaining scorch marks found in his backyard, he said he took a surgery towel and his shirt into the yard and tried to burn them. It was his custom to burn medical periodicals and documents he did not want. The straw on the staircase came from drug hampers, and the children "played at Father Christmas with it."

About the state of the bath he said, "I am a very particular man, and about 365 days of the year I take a bath. The bath was in the same condition it would be after someone had used it. It is nothing more than that. The rest is all this bloody nonsense."

Ruxton was asked if he thought his wife was alive or dead. He replied, "If I may say so, Isabella has done this trick of going to Holland without a passport. If one can do that, there is no limit to what one can do."

One of the interesting subsidiary matters in the Ruxton case concerned the question of the knife or knives with which the dismemberment work was performed. One knife, it was agreed, would have been insufficient for the work unless it were repeatedly sharpened. No knives were found among the equipment in Dr. Ruxton's surgery, and asked in court to explain that fact, Ruxton first said that he had never done major surgery. Pressed on the point, and confronted with his own inventory, he admitted he had had a "slip-on" knife with packets of small blades, but that only one packet had been opened.

Another forensic marginal note attracted a great deal of interest – this was the decision by the prosecution to make enlarged life-size photographs of the two victims and superimpose them on natural-size photographs of their partly-cleaned skulls. The object was to demonstrate that the two victims were who the prosecution claimed them to be, although with so much other supporting evidence at the Crown's disposal this was scarcely in doubt. The experiment was not helped by the fact that the only photographs available of Mary Rogerson were two very small snapshots. But in the case of Mrs. Ruxton, whose distinguishing features were a very long jaw and prominent teeth, the exact conformity of the profile outlines of the face was striking. The results of the experiment were fascinating, but of little medico-legal value. The trial judge said he felt himself in great difficulty in judging the importance of the photographs either way. He told the jury that you might get a false value from a photograph at any time, and you might get a doubly false value if one photograph is superimposed on another. In the event, it is doubtful whether the jury paid much regard to this "evidence."

The trial lasted 11 days, and at the end of it the jury took only just over an hour to find Ruxton guilty. Before he was sentenced to death he thanked the judge for his patience and fairness. As the judge donned the black cap Ruxton raised his arm in a stiff military salute.

After the execution at Strangeways Prison, Manchester, on Tuesday, May 12th, 1936, a friend of Ruxton's produced a sealed envelope given to him by the doctor. Ruxton left instructions that the envelope should be sent to a newspaper in the event of his execution. When it was opened it was found to have been written the day after his arrest, October 14th, 1935, and it said, "I killed Mrs. Ruxton in a fit of temper because I thought she had been with a man. I was mad at the time. Mary Rogerson was present at the time. I had to kill her. – B. Ruxton."

5

TEETH THAT TELL TALES

"In fifteen years I have examined over 11,000 cases, and I have never seen this injury, except in manual strangulation," Dr. Simpson said

Now that dentists keep accurate records of all the patients they treat, teeth are an obvious aid to identification – a number of cases exist where a corpse has been identified solely as a result of comparing its teeth with dental records.

An unusual case where this happened occurred in London in the nineteenth century and concerned an old Irishwoman named Caroline Walsh, who apparently was repeatedly being solicited by her near-neighbours, Mr. and Mrs. Martin Ross, to come and live with them. Walsh had always refused, until on August 19th she eventually agreed to move in with the Rosses, who lived in a place called Goodman's Fields. She took with her her bed, and an old basket, from which she used to sell tapes and articles for millinery. From the moment she moved in with the Rosses, Caroline Walsh was never seen alive again.

What happened was reported to the police by the Rosses' son. He said that on the evening of Caroline Walsh's arrival at his parents' house she was murdered by his mother, who placed her hands over the mouth of Caroline and pressed hard on her chest until she was dead. He could give no reason why his mother should have done this.

But where, the police demanded to know, was the body? "Well," said young Ross, "I saw the dead body of the old woman lying in the cellar of our house the very next morning. And in the evening I saw my mother leaving the house with something large and heavy in a sack."

Then an extraordinary thing happened. In the evening of August 20th – the day following the murder and the same day when young Ross saw his mother leaving the house with a sack – an old woman was found lying in the street in the near-neighbourhood of the Ross house. This woman seem to bear something of a resemblance to Caroline Walsh. She was in an exhausted condition, filthy, and smelt terribly. The police were called to deal with her and at the police station she told them her name was Caroline Welsh, and that she came from Ireland. Before proper inquiries could be made she was found to have a fractured hip, and was immediately taken off to the London Hospital. She died during the operation, and was subsequently buried.

Mrs. Ross, now accused of murder, at once told the police, "But I couldn't have killed Caroline. You found her in the street, took her to hospital, and she died there."

"That was a different Caroline," the police insisted. But could they prove it? For the extraordinary similarity of names and the exact coincidence of time and place must have bothered them a great deal as they drew up the brief to try Mrs. Ross for murder. They dug up Caroline Welsh, the hospital victim, and twenty prosecution witnesses were assembled to establish the points of difference between the two women, despite all the astonishing coincidences. The witnesses testified that both women were indeed Irishwomen, but Caroline Walsh, who had been murdered, was from Kilkenny, and Caroline Welsh, who died during an operation, was from Waterford. The murder victim was 84, tall, sallow in complexion, grey-haired, and had – remarkably for her age – perfect incisor teeth. The operation victim was 60, tall, dark, and not only had no front teeth but all the cavities corresponding to them had been obliterated. To prove the point her skull was brought to court.

Although the two women dressed very similarly Caroline Walsh – whose body was never found – was in good health, and her feet were in good shape. Caroline Welsh, on the other hand, was emaciated and had a broken hip; her feet were covered with bunions, and one toe overlapped another. Although both women owned similar baskets, everyone knew that the one owned by Caroline Walsh had no cover to it, while the one found on Caroline Welsh did have a cover. It was also proved that some articles of Caroline Walsh's clothing had been sold by Mrs. Ross. Even so, doubts would have lingered on – for the coincidences in the case were remarkable – had it not been for the evidence of Caroline Welsh's jaw, produced in court. That was enough for the jury to find Mrs. Ross guilty of murder.

Londoner Mrs. Rachel Dobkin met her estranged husband Harry in a Shoreditch cafe on Good Friday, April 11th, 1941, and was never seen alive again. There was nothing quite as unusual in this as there would be today – enemy action claimed thousands of civilian lives in London, and while bodies were generally accounted for, they were not all accounted for immediately.. Three days later, on the night of April 14th, a fire broke out in the cellar of a ruined Baptist chapel in Vauxhall Road next to the building where Mrs. Dobkin's husband was employed as a firewatcher. (A firewatcher was a person who surveyed the neighbourhood at night from a vantage point, and when during a raid fire broke out, he or she directed the fire brigade by phone to the source of the incident). But on this particular night there had been no enemy action, and therefore there was no reason for a fire. Two hours passed before the fire brigade was called – not by the firewatcher Dobkin, but by a passer-by. There was a heavy air raid the following night, so the incident was soon forgotten.

Fifteen months later, in the summer of 1942, what remained of the Baptist chapel was demolished. Under a stone in the floor of the cellar the demolition workmen discovered partly burned human remains, covered with earth and lime. There was a head, trunk, and parts of arms and legs. In the viscera was a slightly enlarged uterus containing a fibroid tumour. There was also some brown hair, turning grey. All the parts belonged to one body. The head had been cut off, both arms had been severed at the elbow, and both legs at the knee. This of course was no bomb victim – the corpse had been dismembered by a murderer who had started the fire to destroy the evidence.

The Home Office pathologist Dr. Keith Simpson established that these remains were those of a woman aged 40 to 50, and five feet tall. There was a fracture to her hyoid bone, with a blood clot around it, which to a forensic scientist means strangulation.

Even with all the problems of war, the blitz on London and the daily deaths of civilians from bombs raining from the sky, murder was still vigorously investigated. Mrs. Dobkin was 47, about five feet tall, had dark brown hair turning grey and suffered from a fibroid tumour of the uterus. A doctor remembered her from a photograph as his patient; he remembered too that she had refused an operation for the complaint.

Was all this enough to prove that the remains were those of Mrs. Dobkin? Not quite, but the deciding factor was her teeth. The lower jaw was missing, and in the upper jaw there were four teeth only, three molars on the right, two of which had fillings, and the first molar, also filled, on the left. Her dentist, Barnett Kopkin, was called in to describe her dental state: it corresponded exactly with the dental condition of the upper jaw of the remains. Mr. Kopkin's dental records were afterwards described by a police inspector as the most comprehensive he had ever seen. The dentist added that in removing the first and second premolar on the left side he had left a portion of the root. The residual roots were revealed by X-rays to the upper jaw. Shown the jaw, Mr Kopkin said, "That is Mrs. Dobkin's jaw and those are my fillings."

Mrs. Dobkin was Rachel Dubinski when she married Harry Dobkin in 1920 – three days after the ceremony they separated. A daughter was born nine months later, however, and Mrs. Dobkin obtained a court order for maintenance payments. Her husband was wayward with the instalments after the first couple of years, and remained so wayward that he several times went to prison for default. They continued to see each other at irregular intervals, the last occasion being on Good Friday, 1941, when they went to the cafe in Dalston.

Harry Dobkin was arrested and charged with his wife's murder. The case for the defence was that the remains were not Mrs. Dobkin. They ferociously challenged Dr. Simpson on the evidence of the teeth, the height of the dead person, on his assumption that she was strangled. They insisted that Mrs. Dobkin was the victim of bomb blast; Dr. Simpson continued to maintain that no such circumstance resulting from enemy action could have broken the horn of her right hyoid. "I have seen injuries under bomb blast circumstances on many occasions, and the injuries have never been confined to a fracture of the horn, as present here," he said. "In fifteen years I have personally examined over 11,000 cases, and I have never seen this injury except in manual strangulation."

It was telling forensic stuff. So was the pathologist's estimate of the victim's height at 5 feet 1 inch. When the defence put it to Dr. Simpson that if the woman had been two inches taller – 5 ft 3 inches – it could not have been Mrs. Dobkin, he had to agree. A newspaper report was then produced, in which Mrs. Dobkin's sister Polly was alleged to have said that her sister was 5 feet 3 inches. Polly was hastily brought to court. Did she say that? "No, I did not," she said. "Rachel was almost my own height." All eyes followed Polly as she swept out of court after giving her evidence. How tall was she, everyone wondered. They were soon to find out. Triumphantly the prosecution announced that they had just had Polly measured. Without shoes she was a quarter of an inch under five feet; with shoes she was 5 feet 1 inch.

The jury found Harry Dobkin guilty of strangling his wife and burying her body at the height of the Blitz on London. He was hanged at Wandsworth, and Dr. Simpson, the man who sent him to the executioner, performed the post-mortem which is mandatory after judicial execution.

One of the most dramatic murder cases involving forensic science and the study of teeth occurred in recent times when the killer bit his victim's breast in a sexual frenzy and left the evidence that would convict him.

Eighteen-year-old Gordon Hay had his eye on Linda Peacock from the moment he first saw her. Although Linda was only 15, Hay told a friend, "I'd like to have sex with her." That was an unlikely happening. Linda was a bright, lively schoolgirl, interested in ponies, music, and of course boy friends.

But she was not promiscuous.

Why she agreed to a rendezvous with Hay on Sunday, August 6th, 1967, therefore remains something of a mystery. Especially as the rendezvous was at 10 p.m. in St. Mary's cemetery, Biggar, near Glasgow.

It may not have worried her that Hay was an inmate of nearby Loaningdale Approved School for juvenile delinquents because she had once before had a boy friend from the school, and there had been no trouble between them. One of the rules of the approved school was that inmates could not leave the premises after 10 p.m. That didn't worry Gordon Hay. That Sunday evening when he was due to meet Linda he appeared in the school supper room in his dressing-gown and pyjamas, as if to show everyone he had no intention of going out. But after supper he returned to his dormitory and changed into his regular clothing.

He left his pyjamas and dressing-gown on his bed, then slipped out to meet Linda, a couple of minutes' walk away. They were together for no more than fifteen minutes. During that time Hay tied Linda's wrists together, then he hit her on the head, probably with a metal hook he had brought with him.

He didn't have sex with her, but he loosened her upper clothing and for some reason best known only to himself, probably in a fit of sexual frenzy, he bit her savagely on the right breast. If at that moment Linda was conscious she would have screamed with the pain. If she was not conscious, it was because Hay had already strangled her with a ligature he had tied around her neck. Again, for some reason best known to himself, instead of untying the cord he had fastened around her wrists, he burned it off.

Within half an hour of sneaking out of his approved school he was sneaking back again, with his hair disordered and dirt on his clothing.

That night, as the still-warm corpse of Linda Peacock lay under the cemetery yew tree Hay stayed awake, a worried man. How many people knew about his meeting with Linda? How many had seen him with her? At breakfast next day he cornered some of his friends, social misfits like himself.

"Say I was with you in here last night if anyone asks you," he said. For some at Loaningdale Approved School, where a nod was as good as a wink, that was enough for them to agree. But what Hay did not know was that the alibi he was trying to put together was going to be of no use to him at all. For even while he was concocting lies about his whereabouts the previous evening police had found Linda's body, and an observant police photographer was already pointing out the oval bite-marks on Linda's right breast. Those marks were sufficient reason for Glasgow police to bring Dr. Warren Harvey, Scotland's foremost forensic odontologist – odontology is the forensic science of bite-marks – on to their investigative team.

First they had to interview every young man living in the area of St. Mary's cemetery – three thousand of them. All were eliminated. That left only one group, the 29 youths who had been sent to Loaningdale Approved School for their various juvenile offences.

By now Dr. Harvey had examined the distinctive bite-marks in great detail. One mark in particular looked as if it might have come from an unusually sharp and jagged tooth. Whose tooth? To answer that question he would have to have plaster casts made of the teeth of all the 29 inmates of Loaningdale.

When it came to Gordon Hay's turn to have his teeth moulded he was very willing, even delighted, to assist. But like Cinderella's slipper, the cast fitted the bite-mark – and Hay's cheerful willingness to oblige turned to dismay as he was arrested for the murder of

Linda Peacock.

When Hay was put on trial Scotland's Solicitor-General, Ewen Stewart QC, told the High Court in Edinburgh that there would be few if any people with a similar dental structure to Hay's in Britain, or indeed anywhere in the world. And all the times of Hay's known whereabouts on that Sunday, and the times he was missing, fitted perfectly into the crime having been committed by Hay.

Dr. Harvey told the court that he had spent more than 200 hours examining the plaster casts of the teeth of the pupils and staff at Loaningdale. He was able to reduce the number of suspects to five, and then, using a specially designed apparatus that enabled him to simulate bite, grind and slide, he eliminated four of them.

"In the one that remained I found certain dramatic and outstanding features," he said. "In the tips of the two opposite upper and lower canine teeth there were small pits." These pits were like tiny craters, and were symptoms of a rare disorder called hypo-calcination. It was quite extraordinary, the doctor said, to find marks that had a pale centre. "An unusual teeth formation must have caused these marks."

Hay's teeth, he went on, had the equipment to make the wounds. Half of the left central tooth in the upper mouth was broken, leaving sharp edges. He had been able to feel these edges in Hay's mouth.

The tests had been checked with state-of-the-art techniques in dentistry. "I find it extremely difficult to conceive that another mouth could have this number of extraordinary characteristics," he said. His evidence was supported by Dr. Simpson, who said that in 30 years' practice he had not seen any bite-marks with better defined details.

"The teeth made very distinct impressions on the girl's breast and a very firm hold had been taken. That hold was maintained, causing flushing and tiny haemorrhages. This therefore must have been a very painful bite."

He had to admit, though, that there was a problem. The only textbook on the subject in the world suggested a minimum of four or five adjacent teeth corresponding with bite-marks for an infallible identification. In this case there were only three teeth-marks, and they were not even adjacent. Dr. Simpson's case was that the three teeth-marks were so unusual that they made up for the deficiency in teeth. But defence counsel Mr. W. Stewart QC, had already read that one textbook, written by a Swedish expert, and Simpson was at once asked if he agreed with that expert.

"I think it is a sound view," he replied. "But I think a better attitude is a general one – that is to say that the more points of comparison that can be pointed to the more certain the proof, and the fewer the less certain. I would not fix any given number of 3, 4, 5, or 6, but I would say the more you can point to, the more certain you can be of real matching."

He was asked, "Would you agree that the leading experts in forensic odontology seem to live outside Britain?"

Dr. Simpson replied, "I think they have made strides in this field which have preceded those which have been made here, and therefore they have become leaders." Which was another way of saying "Yes."

He had no doubt after examining the cast of Hay's teeth: he was satisfied that the bite-marks on Linda's body were caused by Hay. Cross-examined by Mr. Stewart for Hay, Dr. Simpson said 16 points of comparison were required in fingerprints. Without doubt fingerprints could make it quite clear that a particular suspect was responsible for a crime.

Mr. Stewart: "I don't think that claim has yet been

made for this science of forensic odontology?"

Dr. Simpson: "I think it is very close, if in fact it has not been made. In the first English case the evidence was such that no doubt was expressed about it."

Police Constable James Kinniburgh said a timed run between the approved school and the yew tree under which Linda's body was found took one minute 43 seconds. At a slow walk the time taken was three minutes 10 seconds.

Before young inmates at the approved school gave evidence Lord Grant, Scotland's Lord Justice-Clerk, directed that their names should not be published. A 15-year-old youth said that while the school was in camp the previous year at Montrose he found a large fishing hook in a fishing boat which he took back with him to the school as a memento. Later he showed it to Hay. He showed Hay how to do a trick with a piece of cord, and afterwards Hay put the cord in his pocket. Later that day they went to a cinema and a fairground and saw Linda Peacock. Hay said he wouldn't mind going out with her.

The following day, Sunday, Hay announced his intention of visiting Biggar. There was a whist drive in the school during the early evening, and Hay was one of those present. Soon after it he saw Hay in his pyjamas and dressing-gown, but wearing boots.

Later the youth made a search of the premises but couldn't find Hay. The fisherman's hook, which he had put in his wardrobe, was missing. Hay's dressing-gown and pyjamas were on his bed. When Hay finally came in he was dressed in his outdoor clothing. The knees of his jeans were dirty, his face was dirty and his hair dishevelled. "It looked as though he had been working in the garden and had been kneeling down."

The following morning the youth found that the fisherman's hook had been returned to the wardrobe, and when he told Hay he had been searching for him the previous evening, Hay said he had been in the bathroom. When he asked Hay if had heard there had been a murder in Biggar the previous night, Hay replied, "Was there?"

The youth told the court that he had previously said to the police that no one was out of the dormitory that night "because I was scared." He added, "After I was interviewed by the police Hay asked me about whether I had told them where he was. I said I had told them we were in the sitting-room, and Hay replied, 'That's all right, then.'" Immediately after the murder the youth was not prepared to say anything that would implicate Hay, but he later changed his mind.

The Deputy Headmaster of the approved school, Clifford Lloyd Davis, admitted that occasionally "boys sneaked out to meet girls," though this was not a common occurrence. There was more flexibility in carrying out rules on Sundays than on other days.

A former pupil giving evidence about the whereabouts of Hay on the night of the murder, was told on several occasions by Lord Grant to confine himself to answering the questions. "Please look at me when I am asking you questions," Lord Grant told him. Both this witness and another former inmate of the school admitted that in the witness room there had been a discussion among the boys who were to give evidence as to the time at which certain events took place on the night of the murder. One witness said there had been a discussion "about getting their times right."

Hay told the court, "The only time I was out during the day was up to the football field to play football. After I came down, I was never out of the school at all." After the whist drive on Sunday evening he changed from his day clothes into pyjama trousers, a white casual shirt, and boots. He had supper about

9.30 p.m. and then watched *The Untouchables* in the television room. Just before 10 p.m. he went into the dining-room, where he watched three people playing cards and stood talking to some of them until 10.25 p.m. He went to bed about 10.30 p.m. He had been sent to the approved school, he said, after being convicted of breaking into a factory. He had never been convicted of any offence of assault.

The jury were out for two and a half hours before finding Hay guilty – a significant triumph for the comparatively new forensic science of odontology. Because he was under 18 when he killed Linda, he was sentenced to be detained during Her Majesty's pleasure.

6

CUTTING UP THE BODY

*"In a large square biscuit tin I found one ovary
containing a yellow substance, which is
characteristic of pregnancy," Sir Bernard Spilsbury
told the court*

Patrick Herbert Mahon was a strikingly handsome
man with a ready and charming smile that could
have an equally devastating effect on a susceptible
young girl or a lonely unmarried woman past her
prime. And Mahon knew it. That was why he had
devoted the last fourteen years of his life to the
relentless pursuit of women, all of whom were totally
deceived by his comforting and reassuring manner,
which gave them the feeling they were in safe hands.
In fact, a woman couldn't be in less safe hands than
those of Patrick Mahon, as Emily Kaye was to find
out.

A Liverpool Irishman, Mahon was brought up in
nearby West Derby, and appears to have led a
blameless life until he was twenty, when he married.
But after discovering sex through marriage there was
no stopping him. His first known post-marital
conquest was a young woman he took for a weekend
to the Isle of Man – a trip paid for by a series of forged
cheques. Mahon was arrested, and was lucky enough
to get off with nothing more than being bound over to
keep the peace.

Instead of learning his lesson, he then embarked
upon a career of crime which included embezzlement

and fraud, culminating in robbery with violence when he knocked a girl unconscious with a hammer while he was robbing a Sunningdale bank. By the time he was 34 the good Catholic boy who had been a regular churchgoer had become a liar, a thief and an ex-con who had served five years for robbery with violence.

There is no record of what Mrs. Mahon's feelings were during the time her husband was building himself a reputation for being a violent and habitual criminal. Certainly he wasn't the man she had married. She must have resigned herself to enduring anything to keep the house intact. Loyal to her man she certainly was, and she remained so until the day when she found a cloakroom ticket that was to send Patrick Mahon to the gallows.

When Mahon came out of prison after his five-year stretch he found his wife waiting for him at their home in Pagoda Avenue, Richmond, Surrey. One of their two children had died while Mahon was inside; his homecoming was therefore tinged with some sadness.

But his wife was earning some money. She had a job in Sunbury with a company marketing soda fountains. As a result of her influence Mahon was appointed the company's sales manager. This alone says much for her loyalty, although rather less for the soda company's security control system.

It would now have been quite easy for Mahon to abandon his old ways and become a respectable citizen for the first time in his married life. He had a well-paid job, a reasonable home, and a supportive wife. And for some time he did try. He did his job well, and became a member of Richmond Bowling Club, where he seems to have been well liked by his fellow bowling enthusiasts.

If his job had not taken him to the offices of Robertson, Hill and Company in the City he might well have ended his days in obscurity, contenting himself with the occasional affair until he was too old to be attractive to women. But when he visited Robertson, Hill he met Emily Kaye, a good-looking single woman of 38, who worked there as a secretary. That meeting was to have dire consequences for both of them.

Mahon and Emily were attracted to each other from the start, although he clearly saw her as just another conquest to be discarded as soon as boredom set in. Emily, on the other hand, fell madly in love and saw him as a potential husband, even though she knew he was already married. In no time at all they were on intimate terms.

They had been lovers for some time when Emily decided one afternoon to make her feelings and intentions clear. The place she chose to do this was appropriate – they were in bed in the bed-sit she shared with a woman friend, Eileen Warren, in the Green Cross Club in Guildford Street, London.

"Patrick," she said. "You do love me, don't you?"

"Of course," Mahon said absently, his mind more occupied at that moment with thinking up a new explanation to his wife for his continual late arrivals home. This had become something of a problem – he was sure Mrs. Mahon had already begun to suspect there was another woman in his life.

"And do you mean it, when you say you are no longer in love with your wife?"

"You know that's true." He stared up at the ceiling, his mind suddenly alert as he became aware they were moving into deep waters.

"Then why don't you leave her?"

Mahon sighed. "There's the child to think about, dear."

Emily had decided on the course of action that she considered right for both of them, and she wasn't going to be so easily deflected.

"The child would be better off without you," she told him. Then followed one of those highly charged dialogues which errant husbands often experience, generally ending up with the man promising to do something about it when the right moment came up to speak of divorce.

"Why don't you just leave?" Emily persisted. "We could go abroad. Somewhere far away where she could never bother you again. Somewhere like South Africa. Please say yes, darling."

Lying in bed beside her, with her soft, pliant body pressed against him, Mahon did not have much will-power to protest, although the last thing he wanted to do was to flee to South Africa with her. He struggled to dredge up an objection.

"It's all very well speaking of leaving the country, darling. But there's the matter of finding the money for the fares, to say nothing of the problem of supporting ourselves until I get a job."

"You needn't worry about the fares, or keeping ourselves until you manage to get a job," Emily said triumphantly. "I've got £600 invested in shares which I could sell."

"Have you now?" Mahon said, brightening. Six hundred pounds was the sort of money which in the mid-nineteen-twenties would buy a comfortable detached house in Surrey. "I can see there's no denying you," he said casually. "You'd better turn in your shares tomorrow, and then we can start making arrangements to leave the country."

It is clear that at this stage Mahon had no intention of murdering Emily, but only of getting his hands on her money. Although her nest-egg was a tidy sum for those days, it wasn't enough for him to resort to murder.

Embezzlement or theft, though, were other matters – matters which Mahon treated almost as a way of life.

He didn't have any qualms of conscience about such things.

Why then did he feel impelled to murder Emily Kaye and dispose of her body in the nauseating way that he did? The simple answer was that in due course he was to make a horrific discovery about her for a man in his position. She was pregnant. In 1924 a single woman having a baby was not nearly as commonplace an event as it is today. So when she broke the news of her condition to him Mahon faced what seemed to him an impossible situation.

He hadn't the slightest intention of fleeing the country with her, for that would have meant giving up a well-paid job and deserting his wife and child, a façade of respectability that he had come to value. He certainly wasn't going to contemplate a new life overseas with another young baby to feed, either. On the other hand, if he reneged on his promise to her she would cause a scandal and he would lose his job and become something of a social outcast within the narrow circles in which he had started to move.

For Mahon there was only one answer to the dilemma. Emily would have to go.

We don't know for certain when she told him she was pregnant, but all the evidence produced at the subsequent trial proves beyond doubt that he knew before their arranged meeting in Eastbourne on the fateful day in 1924 which was to be her last. Before that day, much had happened. Emily had sold her shares and had deposited the money in the bank. Then she had drawn £400 and handed it over to Mahon.

In what must have seemed to her a touching gesture of good faith he bought her an expensive ring. Proudly she exhibited it to her room-mate, Eileen Warren, who looked at it with some surprise. For Eileen had met Mahon on several occasions, and he had never once given her the impression of being sufficiently in love with Emily to give up a good job and his family for an uncertain future in South Africa. But she kept her own counsel. She admired the ring and wished Emily well. From then on things began to move fast.

"It's all fixed!" Mahon told Emily one day. "First, though, I've a number of business matters to clear up. Then I'll meet you in Eastbourne. From there we'll go to Paris, where we'll stay until after the Easter holidays. Then we'll go though France and Italy, and from there we'll get a boat to the Cape." He smiled. "You'd better get packed right away. I've booked you in at the Kenilworth Hotel in Eastbourne from the seventh."

Overjoyed, Emily rushed back to her room and began packing. Eileen Warren wasn't there, so Emily resolved to write to her from Eastbourne, apologising for not seeing her before she left, and telling her that if she wanted to get in touch to write care of the Standard Bank in Cape Town.

Arriving at the hotel on April 7th, she duly wrote that letter, and then waited for Mahon, who arrived in Eastbourne on the 4.45 train on April 10th. Earlier in the day he had gone shopping and bought a large cook's knife and a meat saw; now, wrapped in brown paper, they lay at the bottom of his luggage. When Emily came down to meet him at the reception desk of the Kenilworth Hotel he greeted her with an apologetic smile. There was, he said, a slight change of plan.

"As we've plenty of time to catch the sailing to France, I decided at the last moment to rent a bungalow along the coast where we can really be alone. I hope you don't have any objections."

Poor, gullible Emily was only too happy to go along with anything, as long as at the end of it all she landed up in Cape Town with the man she loved. She left the hotel soon afterwards with Mahon and was never seen alive again.

The bungalow, which Mahon had rented under the name of Waller, was known as the Officer's House, from having once been the home of the commander of the coastguard station. It was situated between Eastbourne and Pevensey Bay in an area known as The Crumbles. This desolate stretch of shingle beach had already been the site of a recent murder. Four years previously the body of a young woman, her head smashed in, was found buried in the shingle. Later that year Jack Field and William Gray, both unemployed, were hanged for the crime. Now the same lonely spot was chosen by Patrick Mahon to murder Emily Kaye.

Mahon could scarcely have had any guilt problems while he was taking her to the bungalow, for he had already met another woman with whom he was hoping to embark on yet another brief affair. She was Ethel Primrose Duncan, and he met her on the same day that Emily travelled down to Eastbourne. It was raining heavily, and after striking up a conversation with Ethel and making a few comments about the appalling weather, he offered to see her home.

"It's late and dangerous for a good-looking woman like yourself to be out alone," he told her, his strong, rather prominent jaw giving him the deceptive look of a reliable man who could be implicitly trusted with a woman alone. And such was his extraordinary charm that she agreed to let him walk with her to Isleworth. Before he left her in front of the house she shared with her sister she had agreed to see him again.

They met for the second time at the Victoria Street Restaurant in London on April 15th where they dined together. Earlier that very same day Mahon had murdered Emily Kaye, whose body now lay in one of the bedrooms in the Crumbles bungalow, covered with a coat. She was to lie there for another four days before he began the grisly task of dismembering her.

Over dinner on that evening of the fifteenth Mahon calmly suggested that Ethel should come over and stay at the bungalow the following weekend, the Easter weekend. Although she hardly knew him, she agreed. That was an unwise decision but perhaps it was an all too understandable one. She was thirty-two, lonely, and with little experience of men, and she was completely captivated by the strikingly handsome Patrick Mahon, whose insouciant charm had swept more worldly women than herself off their feet.

So, the following Friday, he met her at Eastbourne station. He was dressed in a smart suit and looked totally relaxed, even though only hours before he had been busy dismembering Emily's body and stuffing her remains safely away in a trunk in one of the bungalow's bedrooms.

What, one wonders, was running through Mahon's mind as he took Ethel Duncan to the Officer's House for that Easter weekend, while the remains of the woman he had just murdered were in the next bedroom? Two suggestions have been made: first, that the weekend with Ethel was a calculated move to allay suspicion; and second, that it was the behaviour of the classic psychopath, impervious to all human feelings.

Ethel Duncan shared Mahon's bed from Good Friday until the following Monday, when they both returned to London. They had dinner and then went to a show at the London Palladium. Afterwards he put her on a train to Isleworth, promising to get in touch again soon.

When Mahon made his way home that night he must have thought he had covered his tracks quite well. Although murder had not been on the agenda in the beginning, he had been careful to hide his relationship with Emily Kaye from his business colleagues, though it had remained a potentially difficult situation until she left Robertson, Hill to work elsewhere in the City. The only person who had known of their relationship was Eileen Warren, and as far as she was concerned the two of them were now on their way to South Africa, a story to which Emily had lent credence with her farewell note to Eileen.

As for Ethel Duncan, she had known Mahon only by the name of Patrick Waller – the name he gave when he rented the bungalow. Although two heart-stopping situations had occurred at the bungalow, he had evaded them easily enough. The first happened when Ethel came across a pair of Emily's shoes and some of her toiletries.

"They must have been left by my wife," Mahon assured her quickly. "She was down here recently."

The other occurred when she discovered him screwing up the door of the bedroom next to where they slept. "The door doesn't lock properly," he told her. "There are some very valuable books in there that belong to a friend of mine. I have to make the room secure."

Ethel accepted this explanation without question. All the same, Mahon couldn't have slept well that night. He still had to dispose of Emily's body, a gruesome task that even he could not have been relishing. What followed next is the stuff of nightmares.

As soon as he had seen Ethel off he went down to the bungalow where he spent all day trying to burn Emily's remains in the sitting-room grate. But attempting to destroy a body by burning it in a fire grate is a formidable task, and by nightfall he had only managed to get rid of the head and the legs. Exhausted, and now in a state of absolute panic, he went home and stayed away from the bungalow until he could steel himself to resume his horrific task. This was not until the Saturday, when Emily Kaye had been dead for more than a week.

When he went to the bungalow for a second time he tried boiling down portions of the body to a slurry which he could dispose of down the lavatory. When he could see he was getting nowhere he set to work on the rest of the body parts like a demented butcher. At the end of it, all he had to show for his efforts were a number of chunks of mangled flesh, some of which he had wrapped up into brown paper parcels and placed in a large Gladstone bag, together with a number of small items and some pieces of Emily's clothing which he had forgotten to burn. When he finally left the bungalow that night, it looked more like a charnel house than a holiday home.

Mahon now took a train from Eastbourne station to London. In those days there was dense undergrowth alongside much of the railway tracks, so periodically he tossed out of the window one of the brown paper parcels with bits of Emily in it. There, he reasoned, the contents would rot.

Still clutching the Gladstone bag, and now unable to face going home, he got off the train at Redhill. There he spent a sleepless night in a hotel. Next day he took another train to Waterloo station, where he deposited the Gladstone bag in left-luggage, intending to pick it up some time before going back to Eastbourne to make yet another attempt to deal with what was left of Emily Kaye.

So far little mention has been made of Mrs. Mahon. She, who had been a constant support to her husband, now becomes a key figure in the drama. What were her feelings about his continual absences from home? He had not put his foot over the threshold of the matrimonial home for two successive weekends and a number of weekdays. What was going on, she must have wondered.

She might not have worried as much as a contemporary housewife would, for in the 1920s a

See chapter 1

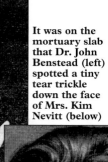

It was on the mortuary slab that Dr. John Benstead (left) spotted a tiny tear trickle down the face of Mrs. Kim Nevitt (below)

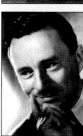

See chapter 4

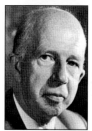

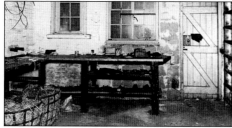

The workshop at Crawley where John Haigh murdered his victims and dissolved them in acid. Above left, Dr. Keith Simpson

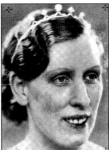
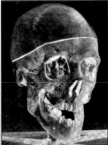
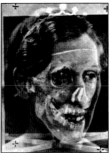

The attempt to identify Mrs. Ruxton (above) and Mary Rogerson (below), by montaging portraits and pictures of their skulls, offered no useful evidence

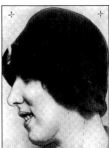
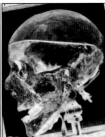
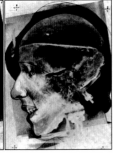

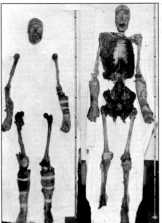

The partly reassembled bodies of Mary Rogerson (far left) and Isabella Ruxton

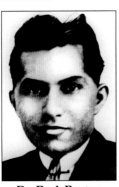

Dr. Buck Ruxton

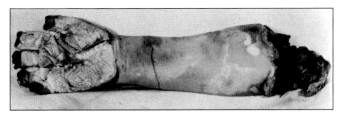

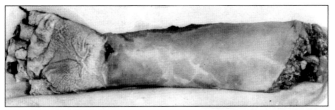

**Mrs. Ruxton's hand and right forearm, and below,
her left forearm. Note the mutilation of the fingers**

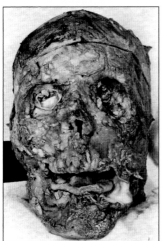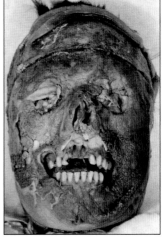

**The head of Mrs. Ruxton with the eyes missing and all the teeth
drawn. Above right, Mary Rogerson's head**

See chapter 4

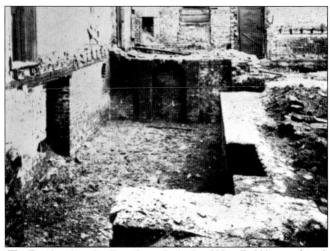

The Baptist chapel cellar where the body of Mrs. Dobkin was found

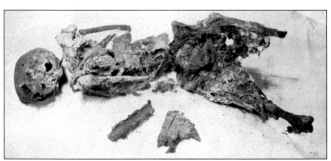

The body as it looked when it was discovered

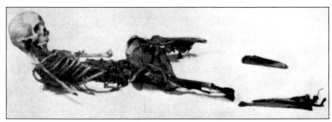

The skeleton after it was cleaned of debris
See chapter 5

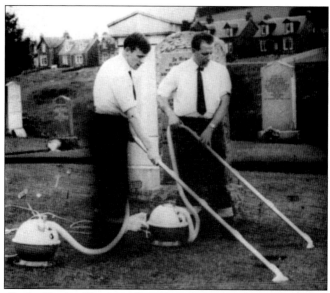

In the Gordon Hay case the entire cemetery was vacuumed for evidence. The case made forensic history being the first time a murderer was convicted largely on the evidence of tooth marks. Below, the casts that matched the bite mark, bottom left

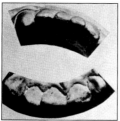

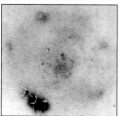

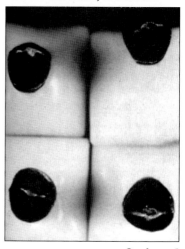

See chapter 5

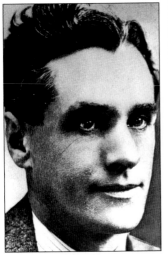
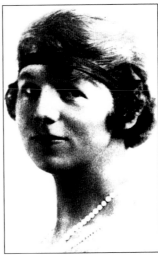

Patrick Mahon and his victim Emily Kaye. Her body and bones were cut into 1,000 pieces. Below, Mahon is led from the murder scene on the Crumbles at Eastbourne

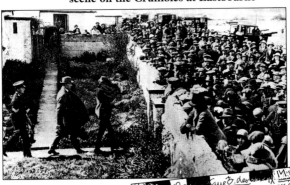

One of Sir Bernard Spilsbury's cards concerning the Mahon case

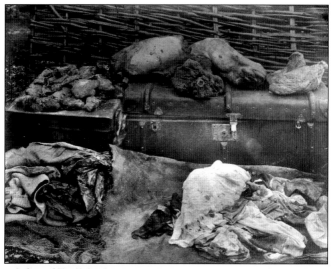

A few of Emily's clothes and lumps of her dismembered body arranged for this police photograph

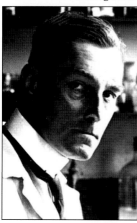

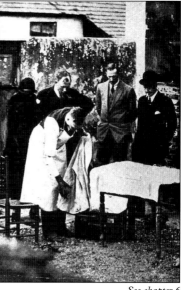

Above, Sir Bernard Spilsbury, and right with his female assistant and police officers outside the bungalow to examine the remains of Emily Kaye

See chapter 6

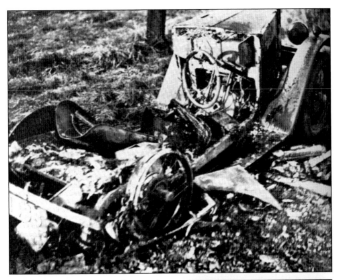

The burnt out car on the road near Hardingstone, Northants. Alfred Rouse (right) thought he could walk away from it and disappear

See chapter 7

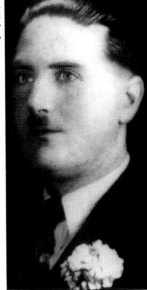

man was considered master of his own home, with the right to come and go unchallenged just as he pleased. On top of that Mahon was a sales manager, a position which gave him an ideal excuse for being away, visiting customers. Even so, Mrs. Mahon knew her husband well enough. Something, she suspected, was going on. To find out what, she had been going through his pockets for some time, but without success.

But on his eventual return from Eastbourne she did find something that set her puzzling – a left-luggage ticket issued at Waterloo station. She looked at the left luggage ticket, the date on it, turned it over in her hand. She was deeply curious. She desperately wanted to know what her husband had left at Waterloo station after coming home from an unexplained weekend away. And she had one friend who could help her answer that question without the slightest trouble – John Beard, a former railway detective. After telling Mr. Beard about her suspicions the two of them went to Waterloo station to collect the bag. It was locked, but Beard could feel a large knife and bloodstained clothing inside. Grim-faced, he said nothing of his discovery to Mrs. Mahon, and returned the bag to left-luggage. He gave the ticket back to Mrs. Mahon, telling her to put it back in the trouser pocket where she had found it.

Then Mr. Beard reported his findings to the police, who unobtrusively hung about the left-luggage boxes, waiting for Mahon to appear. That happened a few days later. At the moment that he went to claim his bag Mahon was arrested. He was taken to Kennington Police Station, where the bag was opened in his presence.

Inside it were a pair of women's knickers and other female clothing, as well as a ten-inch carving knife and a canvas racquet bag with Emily Kaye's initials. All of them were soaked with blood. Asked to explain the blood on the clothing, Mahon said weakly, "I'm fond of dogs. I suppose I have carried home meat for the dogs in it."

"You don't wrap dog's meat in silk," he was told.

Mahon replied, "Dog's meat. You seem to know all about it."

After sitting there for nearly an hour and a half without saying anything more he finally told his interrogators the story he was to repeat at his trial.

Gradually, the story of the Crumbles bungalow murder seeped out. These were the days when a hanging sentence added a dramatic element to a trial which brought the crowds flocking to the spectacle of a man fighting for his life against the machinery of the law. Before Mahon went on trial the press had a field day, reporting what the police had found when they broke into the bungalow.

With morbid fascination the public read about the quartered and limbless remains of Emily Kaye found lying in a trunk, about the heart and other organs discovered in a biscuit tin. By the time the press was finished, Mahon had already been judged and found guilty by most of the public.

Not surprisingly, when he came to trial at Sussex Assizes at Lewes on Tuesday, July 15th, 1924, the courthouse was mobbed by people hoping to get a glimpse of him. There was room for only 200 of them, and as they leaned over the bar of the public gallery they saw a well-dressed young man, above average height, with a pleasant smile. They settled in their seats and waited expectantly.

The court was presided over by Mr. Justice Avory, known as "The Hanging Judge" from the number of killers he had sent to the gallows. Four years earlier he had presided over the trial of those other Crumbles' murderers, Field and Gray. That seemed to bode ill for the prisoner. Appearing for the prosecution was

Sir Henry Curtis-Bennett KC, who was soon to demolish Mahon's feeble defence. Acting for Mahon was Mr. J. D. Cassels, who was one day to become a distinguished judge himself. He must have been well aware that he had a mountain to climb, and after the forensic evidence and the poor showing of Mahon in the witness box, that mountain must have seemed like Everest.

When Sir Henry rose to his feet to open the prosecution he began quietly, but as soon as he got into his stride almost every sentence he uttered was a lethal blow designed to destroy the defence before it had even started. His chief witness was the celebrated Sir Bernard Spilsbury, who was introduced to the jury as lecturer on special pathology at St. Bartholomew's Hospital, London, and honorary pathologist to the Home Office. Spilsbury's spine-chilling evidence was an insight into forensic science that few people, even those working in courts, were aware of, and was to be remembered for years afterwards by all who heard it.

Soon after Mahon's arrest at Waterloo station Spilsbury went with police officers to the Crumbles bungalow. He told the court that in the second bedroom he found a tenon saw which was rusty and greasy and had a piece of flesh adhering to it. He also found women's clothes and a tea-cloth which were blood-stained and greasy and had soot or coal dust sticking to them.

In the dining-room he found a coal scuttle with small blood spots on it. One of its legs was badly dented. A saucer close to the fireplace contained solid fat. Near it was a two-gallon saucepan half full of reddish fluid with a thick layer of grease at the top. At the bottom of it he found a piece of boiled flesh with skin sticking to it. There were ashes in the fireplace and the fire fender was splashed with grease.

In the scullery there was a saucepan, a galvanised

iron bath, and an enamelled bowl, all containing grease, and a hat-box filled with 37 pieces of flesh and women's clothing. Describing the flesh, he said one piece had been cut from the back of the right shoulder and included the shoulder blade, part of the collar bone, and part of the bone of the upper arm. These bones had been sawn across. Another piece of flesh consisted of skin, fat and muscle from the region of the navel. The other 35 pieces of flesh consisted of skin, most of them with fat on them, and many of them with muscle on them. On five pieces of flesh he found pubic hair, fair in colour. All the flesh in the hat-box, Spilsbury said, was human, and all of it had probably been boiled.

He also found a trunk containing four large pieces of a human body, one of the left half of the lower part of the body resembling the pelvis, with muscle and skin attached to it, and the upper part of the thigh bone, including also the lower part of the spine, which had been sawn across. The wall of the vagina was attached to one piece of flesh. On one of these four pieces of flesh he found the breast bone, portions of most of the left ribs, and the right breast.

Sir Henry asked him, "Is there anything you want to tell us about that?"

Spilsbury replied, "When I pressed it, milky fluid escaped from the nipple."

Another of the four pieces of flesh formed the left side of the chest and on the back of this piece he found an area two inches long over the shoulder-blade which had a recent bruise. The left breast was attached to this fragment and had a similar appearance to the right breast.

The four pieces fitted together accurately to form practically the whole of the trunk of a woman, together with portions of the limbs found elsewhere in the house. Spilsbury examined the breasts microscopically. "From their condition I am of the opinion that at the time of her death she was in the early stages of pregnancy."

The bruise on the left shoulder was inflicted shortly before death. "It might have been only a few minutes before death if it was a very serious blow which had been struck, or it might have been inflicted a few hours before death, if it had been of a less serious character."

There were portions of certain organs attached to the trunk. A portion of the right lung was sticking to the right half of the chest wall, and portions of some of the organs of the abdomen were still attached, together with pieces of liver, a small piece of spleen, and one kidney.

"In a large square biscuit tin I found human organs of the chest and of the abdomen in nine separate pieces. One piece was a portion of large intestine eight inches long. Another was a piece of small bowel together with the lower end of the neck of the womb or uterus, which had been cleanly cut across. I found one ovary containing a large yellow substance which is characteristic of pregnancy. The other ovary was missing, and so was the bulk of the uterus."

It would have been of value for the court to have known precisely how advanced Emily Kaye's pregnancy was, but since most of her uterus was missing there was no embryo. Forensic scientists have prepared tables to determine the uterine age of an embryo in a dead woman. For instance, an embryo is one-sixth of an inch long at the end of the first month; at the end of the second month, the uterine age probably reached by Emily's embryo child, the embryo is three-quarters of an inch long. The umbilical cord is a thin thread, the limbs, nose and mouth are evident, the hand has a human appearance. The point about why most of the uterus was missing was never asked at Mahon's trial, nor did Spilsbury ever comment on it. But the reason why Mahon destroyed the uterus first must have been for the same reason he destroyed the head – to prevent recognition. The visual scene of him opening her body and pulling out the recognisable living foetus of his own child, just under an inch long, is horrific to imagine.

From the ashes in the dining-room and sitting-room fireplaces, and from the dustpan in the scullery, Spilsbury collected 900 to 1,000 pieces of human bone. Some of these he fitted together to form the right thigh bone, and others formed the right shin bone. He decided that the flesh could have been cut off the bones by the cook's knife which was found in the Gladstone bag, and the bones could have been sawn through by the tenon saw he found in the second bedroom.

"The skull and the bones of the upper neck were not present in these fragments, nor have I identified any fragments of bone from the left lower limb beyond the point at which it had been severed from the trunk. The portions of trunk, the organs, pieces of boiled flesh and the fragments of bone are all human and correspond to a single body. The four pieces of chest and abdominal wall fit accurately to form one trunk, and the organs in the tin box, together with the fragments of organs attached to the four pieces of trunk, form an almost complete set of human organs. The body was that of an adult female of big build and fair hair. She was probably between one and three months pregnant. The organs were those of a healthy person. I found no disease to account for natural death and no condition which would account for unnatural death. The only evidence of violence was the bruise on the back."

Mr. Cassels, defending, began to presume upon the cause of death as he cross-examined Spilsbury. His questions were to demonstrate that a forensic scientist's job isn't all about blood and bone, it is just as much about observation and deduction. "Suppose," Mr. Cassels conjectured, "there was a struggle in that sitting-room, suppose that in the course of that struggle between two persons a chair was overturned. The two people fell, one on top of the other, then suppose that the under person was to strike their head on a large lump of coal in the scuttle, and suppose at the time of the fall the throat of each was held by the other, would you expect that there might be a wound on the head which would cause bleeding, and that injuries might be received which would cause the rapid death of the under person?"

Spilsbury replied, "No, I should not."

"Why not?"

"Because no fall on to the coal scuttle such as you describe would be capable of inflicting such injuries to the head as to cause rapidly fatal results. In the case of that particular coal scuttle, filled with coal, a sufficiently severe blow to produce such injury would have crumpled up the scuttle."

The inference was already known, because the prosecution had opened by reading out the statement Mahon made when he was arrested. Mahon was going to plead that in an argument with Emily Kaye they fell and she struck her head on the coal scuttle, dying from the injury. But already that argument was torpedoed by Spilsbury's acute observation of the scuttle – a cheap Woolworth's article of the sort a landlord would put into rented accommodation, and so frail that it couldn't kill anyone. At this point Mahon, sitting in the dock, pursed his lips vexedly.

But Mr. Cassels pursued the point. "Have you considered the possibility of the pressure coming from the fall so that the head comes into contact with the coal in the scuttle, but also the pressure which comes from the possible holding of the neck by the person who is on top? What I am suggesting is that you take into consideration the fall, the chair, the scuttle, supplying more or less a leverage, with the pressure of the body and a hand on the neck – would not that have the effect of possibly fracturing one of the neck bones?"

No, replied Spilsbury, it wasn't possible for the neck to be broken in such circumstances.

"The floor probably might cause the injury?"

Spilsbury was unshakeable. "No. If you take a blow which is a glancing one, that scuttle would so far break the fall as to reduce the danger of contact with the floor afterwards."

Mr. Cassels was able to pursue these lines of inquiry because the vital parts of Emily Kaye that could prove him absolutely wrong – the neck and the head – were missing. How Mahon disposed of the head had already been revealed by the prisoner to his defence counsel in an interview at Brixton Prison. He told Mr. Cassels how he built up a big fire in the grate of the dining-room, and placed Emily Kaye's severed head in the middle of it. As the long fair hair flamed up the dead eyes opened. Outside there was a clap of thunder, a flash of lightning. In a state of terror, Mahon said he ran out into the rain. This, of course, was hardly a story that the defence counsel could tell in court.

Mr. Cassels must have found Spilsbury a formidable adversary to his speculation – speculation which, had it succeeded, would have given rise to a lesser charge of manslaughter. Mahon would plead that Emily died accidentally in the struggle, that he never intended to kill her, and that in blind panic he cut up her body and tried to dispose of it. There was nothing much new in that – it was an argument which had been used before by dismembering killers. So the defence went remorselessly on.

"In a fall of that sort, where the coal scuttle had taken a part of pressure and the chair had taken a part, and the body on top might take a part, with its hands around the neck of the body under, you might even get a twist?"

"It is difficult to see how you could."

"Is it to be finally dismissed altogether from speculation?"

"I cannot conceive how it could occur."

"You can only go on speculation?"

"Yes."

"Does it require much violence to bring about such a fracture or shifting of the cervical vertebrae to produce compression of the spinal cord?"

Spilsbury considered the question. Yes, he decided, it did. But it depended upon the nature of the injury. It might be due to haemorrhage or to breaking the bone. If haemorrhage followed the injury, it might appear a lesser injury, and develop very slowly.

Finally Mr. Cassels asked in some desperation, "Cases which you have had of fatal and rapidly fatal compression of the spinal marrow, have they been cases of falls?"

And to the end Spilsbury frustrated him. "I think every case I have had of rapidly fatal compression of the spinal marrow has been a case in which there has been disease of the spinal column." He had already established that Emily Kaye was perfectly healthy when she died, and had no such disease.

Death by misadventure? It seemed highly unlikely after Spilsbury's evidence. Certainly it was the only defence that Mahon thought might just get him off. The problem was, he had already scuppered himself by being in possession of the knife and the meat saw, which he had bought before he went down to meet Emily Kaye at Eastbourne. Once the prosecution had established this, Mahon's defence was in shreds.

But even before that, the jury must have been well on their way to making up their minds that Mahon was guilty as charged. For on the third day of his trial Ethel Duncan went into the witness box. Faced with Mahon again she burst into tears, before giving her evidence in an almost inaudible voice. This was enough in itself to brand Mahon a cold and callous killer, capable of sleeping with her while the dismembered corpse of Emily Kaye lay in the next bedroom. By the time Ethel Duncan had finished Mahon's neck was already in the hangman's noose. All Sir Henry Curtis-Bennett had to do now was to tighten it.

Mr. Cassels did his best for his client. He sent Mahon into the witness box, where he began a long, rambling story of how Emily kept pressurising him to leave his wife. Finally he had agreed reluctantly to take her on a fortnight's holiday, where she would convince him he would be happy with her by a passionate display of love-making. The "love experiment," as Mahon called it, had ended in tragedy when they quarrelled and Miss Kaye attacked him with an axe.

"She leaped across the room, clutching at my face. I did my best to keep her off. We struggled backwards and forwards. She was mad with anger and beginning to get the better of me. I became uneasy with fear, and with a despairing throw I pushed her off, and we both fell over the easy chair to the left of the fire. Her head hit the coal scuttle, and I fell with her on top of her. We were each gripping the other by the throat.

"I think I fainted with the fear and the shock. When I became conscious I saw blood flowing from her head on to the floor. I tried to rouse her. She never moved or answered. I believe I went out into the garden. I believe I fainted again, and when I came back she was still lying there, and dead. I pulled her body into the

No. 2 bedroom and covered it with her fur coat."

His voice thick with emotion, he added, "Knowing that I would be accused of murder, I panicked and decided the only course open to me was to dispose of the body."

He wept when he described to the court how he had dismembered the body. None of this had any effect on the jury. Neither Mr. Cassels's valiant attempts to save him or his own attempts to arouse sympathy made the slightest difference to the outcome of the trial. For the jury had heard Ethel Duncan, and they had heard Spilsbury. And they had also heard the evidence of Eileen Warren, who had sketched in Mahon's early relationship with Miss Kaye, and revealed it to be one based on lies and deceit. But most telling of all to the Sussex jury must have been Mahon's purchase of the knife and the meat saw.

The final speeches were little more than a formality. Mr. Justice Avory recalled a broken axe that had been found in the bungalow by the police. "If that axe were used to batter her head in, that would account for the broken handle, and it would account for the care with which prisoner himself says he destroyed the head of that woman in order to destroy effectively any evidence of the injury which had been inflicted on her head."

The jury took forty minutes to find Mahon guilty. Asked if he had anything to say before sentence, he shouted at the judge, "I feel too conscious of the bitterness and unfairness of the summing-up which you have uttered to say anything except that I am not guilty of murder." When he left the court he looked genuinely aggrieved. A few weeks later, on September 2nd, 1924, he was executed at Wandsworth Prison.

A story is told that on the scaffold Mahon revealed his extraordinary knowledge of hanging events. He had discovered that he had to stand within two chalk marks as the rope was adjusted around his neck. He had also discovered that immediately after fixing the hood over the prisoner's head, the hangman moved quickly to a lever and pulled it, causing the platform on which the victim was standing to swing open. At the moment when he sensed the hangman moving to the lever, Mahon, his feet bound, jumped forward in a desperate attempt to place himself beyond the reach of the trap-door. He misjudged the jump and as the lever was pulled his body swung back and the base of his spine struck the sharp edge of the scaffold. It was that blow, the story goes, and not the breaking of the spine at the neck by the action of hanging, that killed him

Spilsbury later described the remains of Emily Kaye as the most gruesome he had ever encountered. Surprisingly, he followed the case of Patrick Mahon right through to the execution shed. Immediately after the hanging he performed the post-mortem. In execution cases it was normal for the pathologist to open the body of the hanged man at the neck to ascertain the cause of death. But with Mahon's body Spilsbury went much further. He opened the body completely, then spent an hour examining the brain, part of which he took away with him. When the coroner suggested he might be overdoing things Spilsbury replied, "I must do this in my own way."

Interestingly, his notes on the post-mortem on the hanged man make no mention of any injury to the base of the spine caused by the desperate jump, which suggests that Mahon's last few seconds in this world might not have happened quite like that.

7

BURNING THE BODY

"He was the sort of man no one would miss, and I thought he would suit the plan I had in mind,"
Rouse told the police

The case of Patrick Mahon appears in hindsight to have been very neat and simply solved, but at the time of his arrest the prospect of that happening was bleak. Much deliberation was given to how the prisoner could be proved guilty of murder when the victim's head, obviously bearing the murder injuries, was missing. Mahon could of course have been found guilty of manslaughter on the evidence of his own story, and also of attempting to conceal a body, but he would not have hanged for that. Spilsbury's genius was not in assembling bits of the body. He was not able to tell the court from his painstaking work how Emily died – but what he was able to say was how she did not die, that it could not have happened in the way Mahon claimed. That part of his evidence, taken together with the purchase of the knife and the saw before the murder, sealed the prisoner's fate.

Spilsbury gleaned nothing either from the hundreds of bits of bone he collected from the grates in the bungalow, beyond the fact that the tools found in the house were used to saw and cut them, a point which Mahon had already admitted anyway. Nor did he gain any fresh evidence from the flesh melted down in pots. Attempts are made so often to destroy bones by some dismembering murderers that it is almost as if they are aware, as they saw and cut, of the importance of bone recognition to the forensic scientist. Others, as we have seen, simply cut up the body and distribute the parts, with flesh still adhering to bone. Still others leave the pieces in the sort of places where they are not likely to be discovered, and hope that nature will do the rest, even to commencing the disintegration of the bones.

In cases where a skeleton only is dug up, an important question for the forensic scientist is, how long has it been buried? A rough calculation can be made from the amount of marrow, if any, in the interior of the bones, and by the firmness, brittleness, dryness and lightness of the bones. But if the bones have been buried where they are not affected by chemical changes caused by such things as moisture, minerals in the soil or the action of air, as for example, in lead coffins or vaults, they can last in a good state of preservation for hundreds of years. In 1868 the skeleton of the Norman king William Rufus, son of William the Conqueror, was found in near-perfect condition in Winchester after nearly eight centuries' burial. And a story is told that a royal party went into the vaults of St. George's Chapel, Windsor, late one night in the early nineteenth century and dislodged the lid of a vault. Inside the vault the complete human form of King Henry VIII was revealed by the light of a lantern, in a perfect state of preservation after nearly three centuries' burial. The spectacle did not last – a few seconds after air entered the opened vault the skin on the dead king's face collapsed.

When a skeleton is found the bones are sometimes in a heap, caused by changes in the structure of the grave. The forensic scientist's first job is to lay them out in proper order. He can then estimate the height and sex of the dead person. To obtain the height he measures the assembled skeleton and adds an inch to an inch and a half for the thickness of the disintegrated tissue. Even if only one long bone is left the height can be calculated arithmetically by using Pearson's tables – a formula devised by Karl Pearson in 1899, and other formulae developed since then. Sex can be determined particularly by the shape of the pelvis. The bones of the male pelvis are rougher and larger than those of the female and the posterior extremity curves down more steeply to its termination. In the long bones the joint surfaces are usually greater in the male, even when comparison is made with a female of equal height.

The skull is an important aid to determining age at death. We are born with sutures, seen as wiggly lines, on our skulls, which gradually close up as we get older. The order of their closing is predetermined, so that a skull will give an indication, within a margin of 10 years, of the age of its owner when he died.

One favourite way of destruction used by killers determined to efface all recogniseable features of their victim is by burning. The subject of burning bodies covers many pages in the lexicon of forensic science. Burning alive is a horrific death, not much favoured by suicides. A burned body presents a gruesome sight; recently burned, it also presents a stench of charred flesh that lingers in the memory. The human body contains 72 per cent water which gives to the soft structures a power of resisting burning. It also contains an average of five per cent fat, which tends to increase combustibility. Add a dead body to something else which is combustible, such as a mattress or a wooden bed, and you have all the material for fire. In an intense fire, which might become extinguished before the discovery of the body, there would be very considerable destruction.

Bones which have been burned often undergo calcination, which completely alters their constitution.

The shape remains the same, but if burning takes place in the open air the bones will be white; if the burning takes place in a closed fire they will be black or ash-grey. The bone becomes brittle, is easily pulverisable, and dissolves in hydrochloric acid, leaving, if perfectly calcined, only some charcoal but no animal matter.

When the bone can't be any longer recognised by its shape as a bone, the forensic scientist knows that a large quantity of phosphate of calcium in the fire ash suggests that bones were present – this distinguishes the ash of bone from the ashes of other substances. But at this level of disintegration it is not possible to tell whether the bone ash was that of a human or an animal – the precipitin test does not work with bone ash.

That almost all of a human body can be destroyed fairly rapidly in intense heat was demonstrated when a man named Barton, who was a fireman employed at a coal-mine near Wigan, went missing from his work in 1863. Signs of blood around the opening of a steam furnace and some bits of burned clothing known to have been worn by Barton suggested, with other facts, that he had been murdered and pushed into the furnace. A pathologist examined the ashes of the furnace and found portions of skull bone, the roots of two teeth, a couple of pieces of vertebrae, a small portion of arm bone and a small portion of a thigh bone. The intense heat in the furnace had destroyed the internal structure of the bones, but the shape of them was still in evidence. Scientific examination of the clinkers in the furnace revealed the presence of blood. The presumption was that these scanty bits of human were all that was left of Barton – it had taken only eight hours of fierce heat to reduce his body to these few parts.

An extraordinary experiment in the effect of fire on

a body was conducted in America in 1906 during a murder investigation. The story began when a young man named Wenzel Kabat made an offer of $18,000 cash for the farm of Michael McCarty in Wisconsin. McCarty had been neglecting his farm and wanted to sell so that he could marry his fiancée, a town girl who did not relish spending the rest of her life in the country. The deal was struck, the deeds were produced, signed and transferred to Kabat, and McCarty moved off to the town where his girl friend lived.

Or so everyone thought. But after several weeks, when it was discovered that McCarty's fiancée had run off with another man and McCarty himself seemed to have disappeared off the face of the earth, an anxious friend went to the police. A routine check was made on the farm, now owned by Kabat, and when police spoke to the neighbours they found them much impressed by the new owner's zeal and industry. The first day he was there he burned a brush pile that had been cluttering up the place for more than a year. He cleaned up the farm, removing accumulated rubbish and burning it, so that there was a big fire for two days and one night. Local housewives were so impressed that they told their husbands they might take an example from Kabat and begin a clean-up drive.

When the District Attorney was informed of this he pointed out that it was possible that Michael McCarty never left his farm alive. "If Kabat killed McCarty he could have a fine farm without paying for it – the murder would be worth $18,000 as well as the farm to him. We have no solid proof that anyone saw McCarty after the night he was supposed to have sold his farm, and that fire Kabat built sounds really interesting."

The DA and the detectives arranged a little ruse. A police officer called on Kabat and took him down to police headquarters for routine questioning. Then Deputy Jim McGregor and another deputy moved in and started sifting through the remains of a large fire behind a barn with screens of various mesh. After two hours they had collected several pieces of bone, a blackened and bent belt buckle, and half a dozen teeth that appeared to be human. They also gathered a few overall buttons and a fragment of a man's shoe.

"I guess this is where poor old McCarty wound up," McGregor said. "The only good thing you can say about it is that he never learned that his sweetheart was running out on him."

Before they had finished the work Kabat returned from police headquarters and strolled back by the barn.

"What are you fellows up to?" he asked.

"We've been finding some bones in this ash heap," McGregor said. "We reckon they're Mike McCarty's bones."

For a long moment Kabat stared at them speechlessly. Then he burst out laughing.

"You must be figuring I've done away with McCarty," he chuckled.

"That's right. What's so funny about that?"

"What's funny is that you're mistaken. You see, there were pigs' feet and other parts of animals in that fire. McCarty left a lot of junk around after butchering, and I got rid of it."

"These teeth never came from a pig," the deputy retorted. "And what about these overall buttons?"

"I found two pairs of worn-out overalls and three pairs of rotting shoes in an upstairs room, along with a load of other junk. I threw it all on the fire."

Kabat seemed much more amused than annoyed about the whole affair, but his good humour began to evaporate when he was told he was being taken in for questioning. As he was driven back to police headquarters the deputies continued to sift the ashes. They hoped to find a skull, but all that came to light was a few more fragments of bone. They searched the entire farm, looking for places that had been recently dug, but found nothing. They questioned Kabat's farm labourer, Steve Rumley, who said the brush pile had been there for nearly a year and McCarty used to throw all kinds of rubbish on it. "I tossed some feet from butchered pigs into it myself a few months ago," he added.

It didn't seem as if they had a case until they sent the deeds of the farm sale to a handwriting expert, who declared that McCarty's signature was a forgery. Kabat was arrested on a forgery charge, and then news came in that the bits of bone recovered from the ashes, and sent to a Chicago forensic laboratory for examination, were all from a human body.

Even so, this was far from a cut and dried case. For one thing, American juries at this time early in the twentieth century were still sceptical of scientific evidence. For another, lawyers had to admit that even if it was accepted that these were human bones, there was still no actual proof that murder had been committed. How could it be proved that they were the bones of McCarty, or that Kabat had murdered him? As for Kabat, he scoffed at all the murder talk.

"I bet McCarty is alive and well and not far away right now," he declared. Furthermore, he was adamant that a brush fire could never have consumed so much of a human body, leaving not even the skull. In that view he was certainly supported by some scientists.

The prosecutor was now in a tough spot. He was certain a murder had been committed, yet he doubted his ability to prove it in court. And in court, too, there would be some difficult questions asked by the defence about the continued failure to find McCarty's fiancée and the man with whom she had run off.

As the weeks and months passed Kabat, through his lawyers, demanded to be tried. The prosecution continued to ponder how they might prove that the complete body of a man, even his skull, would be consumed if it were burned for two days. If that were not so, how much of it would be left? To try to prove the point one way or another, they called in a Chicago forensic pathologist, Dr. John Golden. After studying the case Dr. Golden proposed a weird experiment to be conducted in strictest secrecy.

The unclaimed body of a man from the Chicago morgue would be taken to an out-of-doors fire and burned on brush identical with Kabat's fire, for the same length of time – 32 hours. The ashes would then be examined to see what was left. If a considerable portion of the skeleton or skull remained, then the state had better give up its murder case against Kabat. However, if what was left was reasonably similar to what was found in the ashes of Kabat's fire, then the state's case would have scientific support.

The plan having been agreed, a large brush fire was built at the Kabat farm under conditions precisely like the previous one. The farm labourer Rumley was on hand to ensure that it was the same, and bystanders and newsmen were kept away. The unclaimed body was clothed just as McCarty had been, and was put in the roaring blaze. After 32 hours the fire was doused and the ashes were sifted in the same manner, by the same deputies.

They found no skull, nor any large sections of skeleton. What they did find was a handful of small, charred bone fragments, five teeth and a few buttons. This was identical to what was found in Kabat's fire. They had proved that a human body could be almost totally consumed in such a blaze.

Kabat was indicted for murder. Then dramatically the mystery of McCarty's missing fiancée was cleared up. She was found dead with her new lover in a cheap hotel in Buenos Aires. A nearly empty bottle of whisky was found on a bedside table, along with a note which said, "Sorry, but this seems the only way out." It turned out that it was mere coincidence that Michael McCarty happened to have disappeared at the same time as his girl friend.

When Wenzel Kabat went for trial on Saturday, June 9th, 1906, lawyers watched the case with interest. Those of them who did not know about the prosecution's extraordinary experiment thought there was little chance of a conviction.

The state witnesses included a handwriting expert and a bone expert. Kabat had a previous conviction for forgery which was brought to the jury's attention, together with evidence that McCarty was never seen alive after meeting Kabat to discuss the sale of the farm.

It was apparent that the defence thought that this was all the prosecution had to offer. The defence lawyers tore into the scientific evidence, claiming it was impossible that a human body could be almost entirely destroyed in the kind of fire that Kabat had built. They called an expert witness to support this view. He insisted that at the very least a large part of the skull and considerable parts of the skeleton would resist the flames.

This was just what the prosecution was hoping for. Dr. Golden was now produced as a surprise witness. The courtroom was stunned as he told of his experiment with an unidentified body brought from Chicago. The bones and teeth recovered from his fire were placed side by side with those recovered from Kabat's fire. The jury could see that they were almost identical; that the main contention of the defence was disproved before their eyes.

Kabat was found guilty of first-degree murder. As

Wisconsin had no capital punishment he was sentenced to life imprisonment. He went to jail still claiming that he was the innocent victim of circumstantial evidence. "If it hadn't been for my previous conviction for forgery I'd be a free man today," he said.

He was assigned to work in the tailor's shop, where he became an expert tailor. He seemed able to turn his hand to anything with success, and with his pleasant personality he became popular with guards and fellow convicts. In 1914, after serving eight years, he proved his skill in another way: by escaping from "escape-proof" Waupan prison. Somehow he got hold of a couple of hacksaws, sawed away two cell bars, opened a corridor door with a wooden key he had made, and got into the tailor's shop. There he dressed in a suit of civilian clothes he had hidden, then miraculously managed to scale the floodlit wall without being seen by the tower guards. A dummy he left in his cell bed ensured that his escape was not discovered until the next morning, by which time he was well clear of the prison. A manhunt was mounted, but Kabat wasn't found. Two years passed, and he was still among the missing.

A long way away, in Austin, Minnesota, a man named Fred Taylor had meanwhile opened a tailoring and dry-cleaning shop. Taylor was well liked in Austin, not only for his tailoring skills but also because he took a friendly interest in men who had served time in prison. He was known to go out of his way to help such people, even finding jobs for them in local industries. Everyone knew about his philanthropy, even the local sheriff, and everyone nodded approval at his rehabilitation work among ex-convicts.

In 1916, however, the sheriff had cause to think differently about Fred Taylor when he got a letter from Waupan Prison saying that an escaped convict named Wenzel Kabat was believed to be working in or around Austin. A picture of Kabat accompanied the letter. The sheriff took one look at the picture and knew at once who Fred Taylor was. It was with real regret that he went to arrest the popular townsman. Kabat admitted his identity, and made no resistance.

"I figured I'd get caught sooner or later," he said. "I'm ready to go back."

Returned to Waupan, he resumed the prison grind. Cheerful, industrious, he once more became the institution's best-liked inmate. Later he was given trustee privileges. In 1940, when he was 60, he was thought to have served a sufficient sentence and released, and a few years later he died. Not once did he admit to the murder of Michael McCarty.

The burning of the unknown man seems a crude way of demonstrating forensic evidence, but it should be remembered that the science was in its infancy as the new century began, and that scientists can only increase their knowledge about the human body by experiment and observation. Indeed, forensic science and the diligent investigation of the crime of murder has reached its present day sophistication only because in the civilised world we place the value of human life – even one human life – above all other values.

In many cases of burning the body is only partially burned, but this is enough to cause death. Then the forensic scientist must decide whether there are other injuries, whether the victim was burned during life or after death, how long he survived it, and whether there any other appearances to account for death apart from the burning. He will know, for instance, that when the epidermis has been removed from an area of skin the affected area will dry after death, becoming a yellowish-brown patch. For this reason it is possible to mistake a small burnt area for a simple graze. In larger areas, it is impossible to mistake a burn or scald for some other superficial wound. If the lesion is deeper there is generally some scorched or roasted flesh, which has an unmistakable and horrific smell.

Blisters are among the signs of reaction which living tissues show towards burns. If a cuticle is removed from a blistered part of a living body the skin underneath will become very red. But if a cuticle is stripped off a dead body the skin becomes hard, dry, and yellowish. There are exceptions even to this rule, and the forensic scientist must take those into consideration. Experiments have shown that blisters can be produced by burns in dead as well as living bodies. They are produced at a lower temperature in the living than in the dead, and they are of a different consistency. It is by such observation that a forensic pathologist can determine whether burning happened before or after death.

Similarly, it has been discovered that fractures of the skull and bleeding in the cranium can occur after death when the head is subjected to intense heat. Carbon monoxide in the blood, carbon particles in the lungs, and toxic changes in the cells of the viscera all point to the person being alive when the fire occurred.

A victim may die in a few minutes or live some hours after being extensively burned, and there may be little change in the burnt part to show when death actually took place. All that can be definitely said is that inflammation can occur only in living tissues, so if it is present the victim must have survived long enough for reaction to set in.

Most burning cases where the victim dies are accidents – few people kill deliberately by burning, and few commit suicide by burning. In one case on record, though, a woman tried to kill her mentally defective son by pouring melted pewter into his ear while he was asleep. The victim was in horrific pain and his head was violently inflamed, but he recovered. The mother then claimed that the boy himself poured the molten pewter into his ear. In another case a Glasgow woman tried to kill her husband by pouring boiling water over his genitals while he was in bed asleep. He died, but the prosecution failed to prove that his death was due to the actual scalding.

What looks like foul play may look somewhat different when the forensic scientist has studied the victim and the crime scene. In a case in Chelsea police were called to a flat after the postman had seen smoke coming through the letter box. A settee was found on fire. A man was lying on it, badly burned. His head and shoulders were so burned, in fact, that all that was left of him was a crumbling, charred mass. The arms and part of the trunk lay still smouldering over the edge of the settee, with the legs sprawled over the floor. First impressions were that this was a case of suicide that might have gone wrong. Then the pathologist discovered the end of a revolver sticking out of the victim's abdomen, which seemed to suggest murder, since suicides don't usually choose the abdomen as a place to shoot themselves.

But subsequent careful withdrawal of the "revolver" showed that it was a gas lighter pistol. The old man had been trying to light a paraffin lamp with the lighter, and had somehow caught his beard on fire. The gas stove was still on, the paraffin lamp lay in a burned hole in the hall, and the old man had stumbled and fallen on the couch. What was first thought to be suicide, then murder, was in fact an accident. The post-mortem confirmed this – the victim had inhaled soot particles, there was carbon monoxide in his lungs, and vital changes showed in blistered burns on his legs.

It was armed with data such as this that Sir Bernard Spilsbury came to a case of body-burning in the nineteen-twenties that is celebrated in the annals of crime. The perpetrator was Alfred Arthur Rouse, who could claim, as Patrick Mahon claimed, that women were his undoing. Rouse was the terrestial equivalent of the sailor with a girl in every port – a commercial traveller with a lover in every town.

"They make up my harem," he would say conspiratorially to anyone in any teashop who he could engage in conversation. That was close to the truth. There were no fewer than eighty women on his visiting list.

But unlike Mahon, Rouse had only reasonably good looks, for all his arrogance and conceit. He was well-built, with dark, brushed-back hair and a small moustache. His mouth was sensual, his complexion florid, his chin heavy. Whatever a man might make of that combination, it seemed to act like a magnet to women.

Now, in his early thirties, he was engulfed in a sea of female troubles. He had wives, mistresses, lovers, and consequently and inevitably in the 1920s, illegitimate children. Inevitably, too, they brought with them expenses which were crippling him. This was despite the fact that he was making around £10 a week – a good salary for the times – as a commercial traveller for a Midland company that made braces and garters.

Rouse was still a teenager when he married Lily May Watkins. Although the nature of his job meant that she would never see much of him, she was to remain true to him to the end. Soon after they were married, Rouse met a 15-year-old girl in Edinburgh, made her pregnant and a few years later "married" her.

A string of teenage mistresses followed. From time to time one of them, a 17-year-old servant girl, travelled around with him in his Morris car. She had just borne him a second child. At that same time another young girl was lying ill in her parents' home in Gellygaer, South Wales, where she too was expecting a child by Rouse.

As Rouse left the home of the parents of his latest bigamous "wife," Ivy Jenkins, in Monmouthshire, he could feel the tangled skeins he had woven closing in around him. For it was clear that his latest set of "in-laws" didn't believe his story that he was Eton and Cambridge educated and had held a commission in the First World War.

"The time has come," Rouse said to himself, studying the latest set of red figures in his bank book, "for me to disappear." But how? He could change his name, adopt a new persona. But eighty women would take some escaping from – could he ever feel really safe in any town? No, disappearing wouldn't do. He needed to be declared officially dead, and then to escape to a new country to begin life all over again.

As he walked deep in thought down Whetstone High Road, in North London, pondering the problem, a beggar stopped him outside the Swan and Pyramid pub.

"Spare a copper for a cup of tea, mister?"

The man was the same height, the same build, as Rouse. A plan flashed through his mind. Although he was a teetotaller, he said, "You look like you're down on your luck. Come and have a drink."

In the pub the stranger told Rouse all he wanted to know. He had no job, no prospects of one, and he hadn't a friend or a relative in the world.

"I'm going to Leicester tomorrow," Rouse said. "If you'd like to try your luck there, I'll gladly give you a lift."

Another beer and a handshake sealed the deal. The following evening the two men met by arrangement outside the same pub. Thoughtfully, Rouse handed the stranger a bottle of whisky to keep him warm on the journey – these were the days before heaters were standard fixtures in cars. It was Wednesday, November 5th, 1930, and as the Morris chugged towards St. Albans the night sky was illuminated from time to time by a bonfire or a rocket. By these lights Rouse could see that the whisky bottle was now half empty. His unknown companion was slumped in his seat, drunk into a stupor.

In Hardingstone Lane, near Hardingstone village, Northampton, Rouse stopped the car, leaned across the comatose stranger, and strangled him. It was a minute or two after midnight. Then he opened the bonnet, loosened the petrol union joint probably with the handle of a mallet which he then threw into the grass verge, and took off the top of the carburettor. Next he took a can of petrol from the boot, doused the dead man with it, and laid a trail of petrol, which he lit with a match. As the car burst into fierce flames Rouse watched it for a few seconds, then, carrying a small attaché case, hurried off down the road. He was confident of two things – by the time the car burned out it would be recognisable only as his car, and the corpse in it would be recognisable only as being about his size and build.

Arrogant as ever, Rouse smiled to himself. He had just "died" in a car accident – he had just set in motion the perfect disappearing act.

His confidence, though, was to last only a matter of seconds. For that evening two young cousins, Alfred Brown and William Bailey, had gone to a dance in Northampton, and were now footing it homewards to Hardingstone. As they came round a bend in the road they saw the spreading glow of the suddenly burning car. They saw too a man slip out of the shadow of a hedge and come hurrying down the road towards them. He was hatless, which was unusual for the season, agitated and breathless, and carried an attache case.

"What's that blaze?" Bailey asked his cousin.

The hatless man, now hurrying away from them, gasped over his shoulder, as if he thought the question was addressed to him, "It looks as though someone's having a bonfire up there."

While Rouse disappeared towards the main Northampton – London road, the two young men ran to the scene of the fire. Bailey ran to fetch his father, who was the Hardingstone village constable, and the three men waited until the fire died down. By that time another policeman had arrived. Then they discovered, lying across the front seats, the charred human body.

The remains were taken to the garage of the Crown Inn garage at Hardingstone, and four days later Sir Bernard Spilsbury arrived to examine them. As he worked he dictated his findings: "Top of head and vault of skull completely destroyed. Brain exposed, shrunken and burned on top. Skin of face and ears destroyed ... Whole chest wall destroyed in front. Front of heart and lungs exposed and partly burned. Skin of abdomen wall destroyed in front ... Forearms and hands completely destroyed and part of each upper arm; quite half, with charred bone projecting from stumps. Left foot completely destroyed; right foot separated and on running-board of car – extremity destroyed and toes missing. Greater part of legs below knees destroyed, thighs deeply burned..."

The body was that of a male, he decided, a deduction made from what he suspected was a piece of prostate gland. The man had small features, and his height was 5 feet 7 or 8 inches. From the teeth Spilsbury reckoned his age was about 30. From the lungs he deduced that he had worked in an extremely dusty atmosphere, possibly a coal mine. Fragments of burnt cloth suggested that he was wearing a well-cut suit of plum cashmere, possibly with a purple pin stripe, a white shirt and blue tie. There were three pennies in the burnt remains of his clothes. Not surprisingly given the state of the remains, Spilsbury wrote down the wrong cause of death: "Fire in car and shock. No indication of poison. Period of survival very short."

One part of the car not obliterated by the fire was the back number plate – MU 1468. Ownership was quickly traced to Rouse, who when he was at home with his real wife lived in Buxted Road, Finchley. Confronted with fragments of clothing taken from the car, Mrs. Rouse couldn't be certain whether they belonged to her husband. Although detectives had no reason to suspect other than that the corpse was that of Alfred Rouse – for why should it be anyone else? – they continued to make routine inquiries about the whereabouts of Rouse, just in case they were mistaken.

What followed suggested that while Rouse might be adept at burning cars, he could only make a hash of trying to disappear. He made his way back to London and caught a coach from the Strand to Gellygaer, with the intention of visiting the girl there who was giving birth to another of his children. In Gellygaer an acquaintance showed him a copy of the evening paper with the story "Blazing Car Mystery" headlined across the front page and asked, "Isn't that your car?"

"No, it isn't," replied Rouse. "My car has been stolen."

The mistake, of course, was that now he had been spotted he couldn't use the burned-out car as an alibi for his death – he had already wrecked his own getaway plan. In fact he told so many people who knew his car that it had been stolen that he must have changed his mind about disappearing, and was now suggesting that the victim of the car blaze must have been the thief. His behaviour now became very peculiar, so much so that when he boarded a London-bound coach the police were told that the man they wanted to interview was a passenger on it. Thus, on the evening of November 9th, the coach was met at Hammersmith by Detective Sergeant Skelly. Told he was wanted for questioning, Rouse said, "I'm very glad it is over. I have had no sleep."

He began a rambling statement, which he had clearly been working on while the coach was heading towards London:

"I picked up a man on the Great North Road. He asked me for a lift. He seemed respectable, and said he was going to the Midlands. After going some distance the engine started to spit, and I thought I was running out of petrol. I pulled into the side of the road. I wanted to relieve myself, and said to the man, 'There's some petrol in the can. You can empty it into the tank while I'm gone.' He said, 'What about a smoke?' I said, 'I have given you all my cigarettes as it is.' I gave him a cigar. I then went some distance along the road, and had just got my trousers down when I noticed a big flame. I ran towards the car, which was in flames. I saw the man was inside, and I tried to open the door, but I couldn't. I was all of a shake. I didn't know what to do, and I ran as hard as I could along the road where I saw the two men. I felt I was responsible for what had happened. I lost my head, and I didn't know what to do, and really don't know what I have done since."

He had taken the attaché case with him, he said, because during the journey he had seen the man's hand on it when it was in the back of the car. Had he stopped his story there, Rouse might have stood a chance. The police had no real evidence against him. They could prove that he owned the car which had been burned, and they had some expert advice that the fire was caused by "a human agency." But they could not identify the dead man, nor could they establish that Rouse knew him. To this day, in fact, no one knows the identity of the victim. More than 2,000 missing-person cases were investigated without success, after the man was buried in Hardingstone churchyard. On a plain cross over his grave are the words, "Here lies the body of an unknown man. Died November 6th, 1930." The police could not even prove that Rouse was the driver of the car at the time of the fire.

From then on the case against him depended upon a series of statements he made himself. Interviewed at Northampton, he continued to babble, and made another statement which was eagerly pounced upon by the newspapers and, some believe, condemned him even before he came to trial. "My wife is really too good for me," he said. "I like a woman who will make a fuss of me. I am very friendly with several women, but it is an expensive game. I was on my way to Leicester on Wednesday when this happened, to draw some money from my firm. I was then going to Wales for the weekend. My harem takes me to several places, and I am not at home a great deal, but my wife doesn't ask questions now."

In the 1920s that sort of public comment from a married man just wasn't acceptable. Words used to describe him were "loathsome," "a man with a disgusting mode of life," and "a blackguard." Delving into his past, police even found a woman in Paris by whom he had had a child. Against this background Rouse's defence lawyers had to find something that would work in his favour. They chose his war record.

Early in 1914 he had joined a London Territorial unit. Sent into the thick of the fighting in France, he was severely wounded in the head. The injury put him in a military hospital for months, and he underwent several operations before being discharged with an army pension.

One lawyer who analysed the case said, "There seems no reasonable doubt that the subsequent behaviour of Rouse in his abnormal sex life might be attributed in part to this head wound."

At the murder-charge hearings before the magistrates' court Rouse seemed outwardly unconcerned at his serious position. When he came into court his first action was to fold his overcoat carefully and place it across the back of the chair in the dock. Then he would smile and raise his hand in a form of salute to the reporters in the gallery, and bow to the bench. He produced the same kind of showmanship when he appeared at the assizes.

His wife – "too good for me" – took a job in Northampton to be near him during his wait in prison and his trial. All the money she and Rouse had saved went on his defence. At one stage in his trial Rouse asked for aspirins. Mrs. Rouse at once offered a bottle of smelling salts, and when Rouse declined it she left the court and shortly afterwards returned with aspirins, which were given to the defendant.

Two damning pieces of evidence were used by the Crown against Rouse. The first was that brought forward by Spilsbury and Dr. Eric Shaw, a Northampton pathologist. The body of the victim had been burnt almost to a cinder, but strangely enough one tiny piece of cloth in the fork of his trousers had not been burnt at all. The doubling up of the left leg against the trunk had prevented air and fire from getting to it. (This "pugilistic attitude" of the body, as it is called, is often adopted by the dead body as a result of intense heat contraction of the stronger arm and leg flexor muscles. It bears no relation to the position at death.) When the fragment of cloth was examined Spilsbury noticed that it still smelt of petrol. He made two alternative suggestions to the court. Either petrol was sprayed through the car at the level of the seats before the victim's left leg was doubled up by the intense heat – the piece of cloth being protected from air and flame when the leg bent – or Rouse had emptied petrol over the man before the fire started.

But even this evidence was later challenged by a defence witness, who said that it was quite possible that the unknown man, lurching drunkenly as he handled the petrol can, had spilt some over himself.

Spilsbury told the court that the intense heat had caused the right foot to drop off on to the running-board of the car. Asked if the man could have been struggling to get out of the car, but was overcome too quickly by the heat to succeed, Spilsbury replied, "The fact that the right leg was extended beyond the door when the body was discovered points to the conclusion that the door must have been open from the time when the body first assumed that position in the car. I can see no other explanation that would account for it."

The other telling piece of evidence against Rouse was given by Colonel Cuthbert Buckle, a fire adjuster for the government and for insurance companies, who had something of a reputation for accuracy. He demonstrated to the jury how the fire, in his view, was deliberately caused by "human agency," with a preliminary loosening of the locknut on the petrol feed-pipe.

When the defence opened, counter-evidence to that was called by Mr. Donald Finnemore, defending Rouse. A witness who said that in his experience over a number of years this locknut was invariably loosened by fire was cross-examined by Norman Birkett KC, later Lord Justice Birkett, for the Crown.

The cross-examination was noteworthy for Birkett's devastating first question to the expert witness. Some lawyers have since claimed that the question was unfair.

"You are an engineer and an expert in your own view," said Birkett. "Well, what is the co-efficient for the expansion of brass?"

The witness hesitated, pondered, said he did not quite understand what was meant, but in the end he had to confess he really did not know.

"And you, an engineer, and an expert, admit you do not know what is the co-efficient for the expansion of brass?" asked Birkett. It was a fatal question, for it upset the whole weight of the testimony of this important witness for the defence.

When Rouse went into the witness box he was asked to explain the lies he had told the police. He couldn't, but he remained arrogantly assertive. Birkett asked him, "Why did you allow more than forty-three hours to pass between the time of the 'accident' and the time you were taken off the coach, without reporting the matter to the police?"

Rouse's reply was unconvincing. "I have very little confidence in local police stations," he said smoothly. "I was waiting until I could go to the fountainhead. One usually goes to the fountainhead when one wants things done."

"Why did you tell Detective Sergeant Skelly that you felt responsible when he took you off the coach?" Birkett persisted.

"Because in the eyes of the police the car owner is always responsible for anything that happens to the car," Rouse replied. Which was fair enough, except that the accused, who had to embellish eveything, then raised one eyelid and added superciliously, "Correct me if I'm wrong."

Rouse did not seem to understand how his denials

were adding up the evidence against him. He had never told the truth in his life – why should he be telling it in the witness box? The jury must inevitably have had in the back of their minds the story of his women and his 'harem', although none of these things had been proved before them. Equally, they must have asked themselves why had he told all these lies if he was innocent. They had heard Rouse himself say that he drove the car which was burned, and in which a dead man was found. So why all the lies about a car which was stolen?

Coming down to bedrock, the case against Rouse was not too strong, even allowing for his admissions. Mr. Justice Talbot made that clear in his summing-up. After going through all the evidence, he said, "There can be no doubt that these facts create grave suspicions against this man who was the owner of the car, and who drove it to the place where it was burned. If he is an innocent man, he has created a great deal of suspicion by his own folly."

Without all the voluntary statements made by the prisoner, the jury would have been in something of a dilemma. If only he had kept silent... As it was, the jury took an hour and a half to find him guilty, ninety minutes which included a break for their lunch and another break to inspect the burned-out car. Before the judge sentenced him to death he declared, "I am not guilty of this murder." Two of his women were in court and sobbed broken-heartedly when they heard the verdict that took Alfred Arthur Rouse out of their lives for ever.

A couple of weeks later Rouse had good reasons for feeling confident when he appeared before the Appeal Court, claiming that there was no evidence on which he could have been rightfully convicted if prejudice and circumstances of grave suspicion were eliminated. So far as the element of suspicion was concerned, he had no one to blame but himself because of his contradictory statements. But, Sir Patrick Hastings KC told the Appeal Court on behalf of Rouse, prejudice against him arose from the course of the prosecution. His character was blazoned abroad in such a way that anyone who had even a moderate view of conduct in private life must have regarded the man with horror. The suggestion of Rouse's immorality must have influenced the jury, Sir Patrick argued.

It had been put forward by the prosecution – despite objections by the defence – that Rouse, a married man, was living on terms of immorality with at least three young women. His statement about "my harem" must have caused a feeling of revulsion against him, and thereby prejudice was created. There was no evidence of any motive for the murder.

A vague suggestion was made by the prosecution that Rouse wanted to burn his car, with a man in it, so as to leave the impression that he, Rouse, was dead. If this was a plan that would enable him to disappear that obviously became impossible because Rouse spoke to two men while the car was burning. Also, within a few hours he was visiting people with whom he was intimately acquainted.

The case, basically, came back to the fact that Rouse had told lies. Apart from that, the only evidence against him was that an unknown man had been found dead in his car, and the car burned. Everything in the circumstances was consistent with this man having got out of the car to get the petrol can to fill the tank, and then as he got back into the car something happened to cause a fire.

He might easily have pitched forward across the front seats and become insensible, Sir Patrick argued. His death, according to Sir Bernard Spilsbury, must have taken place within thirty seconds of the onset of the fire.

The Appeal Court was unconvinced by this eloquent argument and the appeal was dismissed. Rouse was hanged at Bedford Jail on March 10th, 1931. Before his execution his wife and two of his women went to see him to say farewell. There was something about Alfred Rouse that made women believe in him right to the end.

Was Sir Patrick Hastings right in his view, and was an innocent man hanged? The answer is no, because Rouse, who always had plenty to say for himself, made a death cell confession. Referring to his victim he wrote, "He was the sort of man no one would miss, and I thought he would suit the plan I had in mind.

"He drank the whisky neat from the bottle and was getting quite fuzzed. We talked a lot, but he did not tell me who he actually was, and I did not care. I turned into Hardingstone Lane because it was quiet and near a main road, where I could get a lift from a lorry afterwards. I pulled the car up.

"The man was half dozing – the effect of the whisky. I gripped him by the throat with my right hand. I pressed his head against the back of the seat. He slid down, his hat falling off. I saw he had a bald patch on the crown of his head. He just gurgled. I pressed his throat hard. The man did not realise what was happening. I pushed his face back. After making a peculiar noise, the man was silent.

"Then I got out of the car, taking my attache case and the can of petrol with me, I made a trail of petrol to the car. I poured petrol over the man and loosened the petrol union joint and took the top off the carburettor. I ran to the beginning of the petrol trail and put a match to it. The flame rushed to the car, which caught fire at once. The fire was very quick and the whole thing was a mass of flames within a few seconds."

The Rouse case was an interesting one for forensic

science because it begs the question of what would have happened if Rouse hadn't met the two men on the road – who, incidentally, positively identified him as soon as he was arrested – and if he hadn't gone straight to Wales and talked to people who knew him? Would the police have been sufficiently convinced that the body in the car was its owner, Rouse, and could he therefore have disappeared completely?

It seems not, because Spilsbury was certain that the smell of petrol in the fork of the trousers indicated that petrol had been thrown over the man while he was lying across the front seats, and then ignited. But could the body have been mistaken for the body of Rouse, and could it have then been conjectured that the petrol-thrower may have been a man whom he met and who murdered him? That theory was never put to the test because Rouse blew it by his own stupidity. He seems nevertheless a man who got within a whisker of committing a perfect murder.

Despite the way in which he charmed his women, there was a callousness about Rouse no better revealed than in his prison confession. Not many people could forgive him for that dismissive sentence about the unknown man he had brutally murdered, "He was the sort of man no one would miss."

8

SAVAGERY AND SEX

In the body of the first woman victim, who had been dead for three weeks, the forensic pathologist found numerous spermatozoa in a remarkable state of preservation

In many cases of dismembering, the forensic pathologist does not necessarily provide all the vital clues that lead to a verdict in court. In some cases his medical evidence merely supports what the police have already discovered, and in others his evidence is of no real value to the jury because they have overwhelming evidence of other kinds to help them reach their verdict. Because dismemberers are usually bent on the perfect murder they make elementary mistakes spotted by detectives even before the forensic scientist has moved in to study the remains. We have seen that this was the case with Dr. Ruxton – another such case was the murder of Stanley Setty by swashbuckling Donald Hume. But in spite of all the overwhelming circumstantial evidence, the forensic evidence was remarkable in providing the clue that led to Hume's arrest.

Farmworker Sidney Tiffin knew the Essex marshes, where the Thames and its little tributaries spill out into the North Sea, like the back of his hand. So when he set out in the early morning of Friday, October 21st, 1949, to hunt for ducks in the lacework of creeks around the River Blackwater he was not much bothered by the chilling cold or the clammy autumn fog held wraith-like by the sluggish waters. This grim and desolate place that would be low on anyone's list of favourite places to visit was like home to Sidney Tiffin.

As he poled his punt along a narrow waterway not far from the village of Tillingham he noticed what seemed to be a bundle of rags floating in the water near a seawall. He assumed it was a drogue, the type towed by RAF training aircraft, which frequently flew over the marshes, and he made a mental note to collect it on his way back. The RAF paid five shillings (25p) for the recovery of such articles.

Several hours later Mr. Tiffin returned by the same route, pulled out the waterlogged parcel and saw at once that it wasn't a drogue. As he began to unwrap the felt covering he drew back with a gasp of horror. Inside the bundle was the torso of a man, dressed in shirt and pants, with the arms bound behind the back, and with no head or legs. He quickly drove a stake into the mud, tied the bundle to it, punted frantically back down the creek, and then ran two miles across the marshes to fetch the village policeman.

Next day Scotland Yard detectives were in Essex examining the gruesome remains. They were quickly joined by police surgeons who delicately pared away thin layers of skin from the body's fingers to produce fingerprints.

It is a matter of routine these days for the police to take the fingerprints of unidentified bodies: if the dead person has a criminal record he or she will be quickly traced. Even if the person has led a blameless life the fingerprints are kept in case they come in useful for later identification. The task of taking fingerprints from a corpse where the fingers have already been skinned, burned, or partially destroyed by the action of water (as had happened in this case) is difficult but not impossible. The expert peels off a layer of skin and takes the print from the under-side, which presents a reverse picture of the arches, whorls, loops and composites whose ridges make up a fingerprint. These ridges are now valleys, and the valleys between them are have become ridges. When photographed the ridges appear white instead of black, as in a positive photograph; the valleys appear black. To get a picture of the victim's normal print the expert has to reverse the photographic negative.

Using this method the prints were very soon identified – they belonged to a 46-year-old second-hand car dealer, already on the missing persons list, named Stanley Setty. He was an oddly mysterious character, one of the easy-money men flourishing in London in the aftermath of the Second World War who made a handsome living supplying wealthy customers with the sort of luxuries that were hard to come by. He was born Sulman Seti in Baghdad in 1903, came to England with his parents at the age of four, and drifted in and out of a number of shady business ventures which by the age of 24 had led him to short terms in British jails. Gradually he built up a thriving trade as a second-hand car dealer in Warren Street – a road in central London which was then the recognised centre of kerbside buying and selling. A swarthy, 13-stone brute, Setty became a Warren Street character with his flashy displays of expensive jewellery, silk ties and Savile Row suits.

Most of the kerbside trading was conducted in cash, and Setty never made any secret of the large roll of banknotes he invariably carried with him. He wouldn't hesitate when confronted with a real snip to stand on the kerb and count off scores of fivers and tenners. But in his personal, private dealings he was known as a tight-fisted, mean man. Although there were plenty of people ready to buy second-hand cars in the immediate post-war years, petrol was still rationed.

The ever-obliging Setty had learned to overcome that problem – he could supply customers with any number of petrol coupons, all skilfully forged. In fact it was some forged petrol coupons that brought Setty into contact with handsome young Donald Hume.

Hume, psychopath, layabout, con-man and general drifter, was the illegitimate son of a West Country schoolmistress. He was intelligent, and could be a charmer when he tried. But he was also extremely aggressive, and quick to take offence. During the war he served in the RAF, a career cut short when he flew his Blenheim bomber into another plane while coming into land, killing the other plane's three-man crew and sustaining severe head injuries himself.

After his discharge Hume moved into the wartime black market, selling a brew he concocted called "Old English Gin." By the war's end he owned an electrical and radio shop at 620 Finchley Road, in the prosperous North London suburb of Golders Green. He had money in the bank, and was married to Cynthia, a well-educated divorcee. To all outward appearances he was a respectable young businessman.

But nothing lasted long with Hume. By early 1948 he was broke. He was forced to surrender the lease of his shop, although he was able to retain the seven-room flat above it as a home for himself and his wife. To add to his financial worries there was a baby on the way. It was then, in a night-club near Marble Arch, that he met Stanley Setty.

"We sized each other up," the former RAF officer said later. "We weren't particularly attracted, but we realised we could be useful to each other." As a result, Hume became an agent disposing of Setty's forged petrol coupons. Soon he was back living high on the vine, the life he liked best.

Setty helped his young agent expand his income even further by getting him involved in stealing cars.

These were then resprayed and furnished with log-books recovered from crashed vehicles. It quickly emerged that thieving cars was a line that was lucrative, and one for which Hume was well suited. With his new wealth he took a refresher course at Elstree Flying Club and, still working for Setty, became a part-time flying smuggler.

Cynthia Hume soon learned that she had married a man who was frequently called away on secret business trips. She didn't have time to inquire into them too much, for she was now the mother of a baby daughter.

Although their business ventures were prospering, Hume and Setty didn't care much for each other. On Hume's side the grudge was simply that Setty was the boss. There were frequent quarrels, and the last one was trivial. Setty had just resprayed a newly stolen car when Hume's dog, Tony, raced around the vehicle and scratched it. Mad with rage, Setty gave the animal a vicious kick. Hume doted on Tony, and the dog's squeals of pain turned his owner's jealousy into a desire for physical revenge.

The opportunity he was looking for came on Tuesday, October 4th, 1949. Arriving back at his flat that evening, he found his wife and baby out. But Stanley Setty was there. Having paid a surprise visit, he found the door ajar, and had settled himself comfortably on the living-room sofa, unaware of the animosity that Hume was secretly nursing towards him.

"On your way, or I'll sling you downstairs!" Hume shouted.

"You'll be the one to get slung down," retorted Setty. At that Hume snapped. He picked up a German SS dagger – a wartime souvenir – and he and the more heavily built Setty were soon rolling around the floor in a desperate fight. Hume forced himself on top of

Setty, then plunged the dagger again and again between the car dealer's ribs. With a final hoarse, rasping cough, Setty fell back dead.

With the flowing of Setty's lifeblood, Hume's passion drained away and panic set in. The dead man's car was outside the flat, there was blood everywhere, and soon Cynthia would be back to discover the appalling crime. But Hume's animal cunning quickly asserted itself. He could still get away with murder, he decided. He began to formulate a plan.

His first need was to conceal the body. Heaving and panting, he dragged Setty's bulk through the rooms of the flat to a small coal cupboard beyond the kitchen. He pushed the corpse inside, covered it with a piece of old felt, and closed the door. Next, with cloth, soap and water, he began to mop up the bloodstains in the living-room. He worked fast, until everything in the room shone with its usual cleanliness, except for a stain on the carpet which he could not totally remove. Then he drove Setty's car back to its mews garage, parked it in the yard – having astutely remembered to wear gloves to avoid leaving fingerprints – and took a taxi back to his flat.

Next day, while Cynthia took the baby to hospital for a medical check, Hume dragged the corpse into the breakfast room. Working rapidly and crudely with a hacksaw, he decapitated the body and severed the legs. At the end of two and a half hours he had the remains wrapped up in three parcels: one containing the legs, the second the head, and the third the torso. He stuffed the torso parcel back into the coal cupboard and set out for Elstree Flying Club with the other two parcels.

By three o'clock that afternoon he was airborne in a small Auster plane, on course for the English Channel and with fuel for three and a half hours' flying time.

Over the Channel he pushed open the Auster's door and heaved out the weighted parcels. "I looked for a sign of them in the sea," he said. "There was none. They must have sunk like a stone."

Because he had no night flying licence, he flew to Southend and left the aircraft there, returning home in a hired car. Next day he took his living-room carpet to be cleaned, brought in a man to decorate the room, and, helped by the decorator, got the torso parcel down the stairs to his car. With the lead weights he had placed inside the parcel, this last task was something of a struggle. At one stage Hume slipped on the stairs and heard the parcel emit "squishy gurgling noises." The decorator appeared not to hear them.

With his dog Tony, Hume drove to Southend and once again flew off towards the Channel. But this time the visibility was poor. He could see water but he didn't know where he was. Flying the aircraft with one hand, he tried again and again to tip the bundle out of the Auster's open door. He was worried that Tony might fall out with it.

At last he manoeuvred it into position and gave it a hefty shove, but with frightening results. As it tipped away into space the felt coverings became partly unwrapped, and the weights which were to carry the evidence to the seabed spilled out. Hume watched the parcel splash into the water and then bob along the surface. All that he could now hope for was that the tide would carry the corpse away and dispose of it. But the tide was against him. On its flood it carried the headless torso landwards, through the River Blackwater, and into the narrow creek where Sidney Tiffin found it. And once the police had identified the torso the missing limbs turned up on the tide.

Forensic pathologist Dr. Francis Camps, examining the body, now provided the clue that was to lead to Hume. He considered that because every bone in the body was broken, it must have been dropped from a great height, which suggested a plane. Enquiries were made at the airports around London, and one of the Elstree mechanics recalled helping a pilot carry two large parcels on to an Auster on the afternoon of October 5th. The plane had returned to Southend that same evening, minus the two parcels, and next day the pilot came back with an even heavier parcel. He took off and later landed at Gravesend field. He then returned to Elstree without the parcel.

Hume was traced to his flat, and charged with murder. He was put on trial on Thursday, January 19th, 1950. The prosecution's medical evidence was in the hands of Francis Camps and Professor Donald Teare. Camps said the cause of death was shock and haemorrhage from five stab wounds. Setty was killed, he thought, about 48 hours before the body was recovered from the sea. The blood on Hume's carpet, he reasoned, must have been Setty's.

The court began to consider the question whether, because of Setty's great bulk, Hume could have killed him on his own. Mr. R. F. Levy QC, prosecuting, asked Dr. Teare if he thought that Setty was possibly killed by more than one assailant. Teare took a long time before replying that because there were no marks on the body caused by Setty defending himself, he was probably killed by more than one person. This evidence is interesting because it shows that even experts can be very wrong. After the trial Hume made a full confession – he had no accomplice.

Teare and Camps were unable to agree about the struggle in Hume's flat that resulted in Setty's death. Camps thought Setty's desperate fight for life would have been very short and very quiet. Teare thought there would have been considerable resistance from Setty. "I should expect a volume of blood to be coughed up, which would be distributed over the assailant." But there would not be much blood from the wounds – a seeping rather than a spurting. Both experts agreed that the total loss of blood would be between three and five pints – enough to have given Hume a considerable cleaning-up problem.

Hume's case was that he was doing a bit of harmless smuggling for a couple of villains, and had no idea what was in the parcels, which he had been asked to dispose of for a total of £200. He was quite unrepentant about his activities on the fringes of crime, freely admitting he had always been prepared to fix up his clients with forged petrol coupons whenever necessary. "Rather than refer to me as an honest man, it would perhaps be better to call me a semi-honest man," he smiled.

With the benefit of hindsight, it seems astonishing that neither police investigation nor forensic science could provide enough evidence to find Hume guilty. The obvious target should have been the cleaned carpet and the bloodstained flat – it is hard to believe that none of the bloodstains found there could be tested positive. When it came down to it, the case against him was purely circumstantial, and his story was further strengthened when Mrs. Hume was called to give evidence.

"Would it have been possible for your husband to have murdered Setty in the flat without your knowledge?" she was asked by defence counsel.

"It would have been quite impossible," she answered firmly.

"Did you see any signs of blood anywhere?" she was then asked. "Or stained knives, or anything like that?"

"None at all."

The daily help, a Mrs. Stride, reinforced Cynthia Hume's evidence.

"I arrived at the flat at about 2 p.m.," she told the court. "I did notice the carpet was missing, and when

I commented on that Hume told me he had put it away in preparation for him staining the floor." He then told her he was going upstairs to clean out some cupboards, and in no circumstances was he to be disturbed. For the rest of the afternoon she heard no unusual noises in the flat, nor saw any bloodstains or signs of a struggle anywhere.

The jury, after a rambling summing-up by the judge, seemed to be thoroughly confused, and eventually announced that they were unable to agree on a verdict. A new jury was empanelled. They were informed by the judge that a verdict of Not Guilty should be brought in for the murder charge, but that he would accept a plea from Hume of being guilty of an accessory charge. Hardly able to believe his luck, Hume changed his plea, and was sentenced to twelve years' imprisonment.

After serving just over eight years he was released, and made a full confession to a Sunday newspaper in return for a considerable sum of money. He then turned bank robber, gunning down a cashier as he robbed the till. With the police hot on his trail, he fled to Switzerland and robbed a bank there, wounding a cashier in the process. As he fled into the street a taxi-driver tried to stop him; Hume shot and killed him with a bullet in the chest. He was caught, jailed for life, and in 1976 he was judged to be insane and was returned in chains to Britain, where he was confined in a hospital for low-risk patients. He died a few years ago.

The extraordinary serial killer John Christie did not cut up the bodies of his victims – he kept them for future reference at his flat in 10 Rillington Place, London, and thereby created a whole new data bank of specimen information for forensic scientists. A new tenant who took over the flat discovered an alcove cupboard hidden under wallpaper, and when he opened it up he found three women sprawled in a heap on top of a pile of rubbish. All three were half-naked and dead.

Dr. Francis Camps was just sitting down to dinner when he was called by the police. He decided that all three women had been partly gassed before they were strangled. The first body was attached by the bra straps to the second body. The third body, wrapped in a blanket, was tied at the ankles. All three were women in their twenties and had died at different times. Although dead from periods ranging between 17 to 64 days, they were still quite pink externally, a characteristic sign of carbon monoxide poisoning. There was no bloodstained fluid from the mouths or in the air passages, which confirmed the absence of decomposition in the lungs. Ripping up the floorboards, the police discovered a fourth body – that of Christie's wife, Ethel, aged 53. She had been dead for several months.

Driven on by this new find, they dug up the garden, uncovering the skeletons of two women. Camps determined that they had been sexually assaulted and strangled about ten years previously. The head of one of the skeletons was missing. Preliminary examination showed that a dustbin had been used as an incinerator to cremate one of the bodies, and that afterwards the whole "casket" of ashes and charred bones was buried.

A tobacco tin found in Christie's bedroom contained four different sets of pubic hairs, all taken from the bodies of four different women. So here clearly was evidence of sexual deviancy, and as Camps began to study the three bodies found in the kitchen cupboard he knew where to look for support evidence. In the vagina of the first body, that of Hectorina MacLennan (who had been dead for about three weeks) he found numerous spermatozoa, complete with tails and in a remarkable state of preservation. In the second body, Maloney, who had been dead for at least two months, there were also fresh spermatozoa. In the third body, Rita Nelson, which had been dead a little longer than the second, there were more spermatozoa, but they were degenerating. From rape cases it is known that spermatozoa degenerate fairly rapidly in a living female, but this is helped by natural drainage. The only explanation for their presence in the three corpses was that the bodies must have been subjected to sexual intercourse after death – necrophilia. The reason the three corpses were reasonably well preserved was brought about by the constant circulation of air within the cupboard.

Some of the people gathering outside 10 Rillington Place in the next few days remembered that four years earlier the tenant of the top floor flat, Timothy John Evans, had been tried for the murder of his 19-year-old wife Beryl and their daughter Geraldine, aged 11 months. The method of concealment was similar – in a cupboard by the sink in a wash-house at the back of the house. Evans, who had a mental age of 10, was tried, found guilty, and hanged at Pentonville in 1950. Two murderers living in different flats at the same house? Was it possible?

John Christie was arrested while leaning against a wall on the Thames Embankment near Putney Bridge. He willingly told detectives the incredible tale of 10 Rillington Place. He met his first victim, Ruth Fuerst, an Austrian prostitute, in the summer of 1943 while his wife was away in Sheffield. He took the girl home and while they were having intercourse he strangled her with a piece of rope. Later he burned her body in the garden.

In December, 1943, he met Muriel Eady, a factory worker. She came to his house once by appointment, complaining of catarrh, which Christie, a first-aid expert, had said he could cure.

"I think I mixed up some stuff, some inhalants – Friar's Balsam was one. She was in the kitchen, inhaling with a scarf over her head. The inhalant was in a square glass jar with a metal screw-top lid. I had made two holes in the lid and through one of the holes I put a rubber tube from the gas bracket on the wall into the liquid. The idea was to stop what was coming out smelling of gas. She inhaled the stuff from the tube. I did it to make her dopey. She became sort of unconscious, and I have a vague recollection of getting a stocking and tying it round her neck. I believe I had intercourse with her at the time I strangled her. I think I put her in the wash-house. That night I buried her in the garden. She still had her clothes on."

Eight years later Christie killed his wife because, he claimed, she was having convulsions. He could not bear to see her in that state, so he got a stocking and put it round her neck "to put her to sleep."

He gassed the three women found in the kitchen alcove by getting them to sit in a deck-chair which he kept in the kitchen between the table and the door. The gas pipe was on the wall next to the window. He put a piece of rubber tubing over the pipe, letting it hang down nearly to the floor.

"When they sat in the deck-chair with the tube behind them I just took off the clip and let the fumes rise from the back of the deck chair. When they started getting overcome, that's when I must have strangled them."

Christie would thus appear to have given a comprehensive account of his killings, but because any statement made by an accused person must be regarded as suspect, corroborative evidence – in this case in the form of forensic evidence – must be included in the prosecution's case. Dr. Camps found carbon monoxide in each of the bodies that Christie said he had gassed. The reaction of his victims to it as described by Christie was consistent with the known facts – people who are being poisoned by carbon monoxide show lassitude, faintness, nausea, loss of power, coma and finally death. Christie's claim that he strangled them to bring about death was also supported by the medical evidence. Unconsciousness would have resulted in a victim sitting in the deck-chair by the time their blood was still less than 50% saturated with gas, a process which would take about a quarter of an hour. Dr. Camps was able to show that in the case of MacLennan, carbon monoxide saturation in her blood was 36%; with Maloney it was 40%, and with Nelson it was 34%.

Camps wondered, though, why the three women whose bodies were found in the alcove had not heard the hissing sound that the escaping gas would have made, and why they hadn't noticed the smell. Possibly, it was thought, there was some sort of canopy over the chair. Another question was, why hadn't Christie himself been affected by the escaping gas? His own answer was that he was standing by an open window. Dr. Camps thought that was "not very satisfactory" as an answer. "If it is assumed that as soon as the victim lost consciousness he turned off the gas and then had intercourse, he might, by taking exercise, have built up a sufficiently high concentration to make himself unconscious. If he opened the window after gassing the victim then the concentration in the air would diminish and the victim begin to recover, but it seems possible that his own saturation might have been too high for him to carry out any active business in comfort. It is possible that it could have happened as he said, but improbable unless Christie himself was using some protection or was outside the room at the time (which he denied)." All such points had to be examined and forensically tested, particularly in a case like this, where the prisoner was claiming to be as mad as a March hare and seeking to gain a life sentence in a mental asylum as a preferable alternative to a date with the hangman.

John Christie was tried at the Old Bailey for only one murder – that of his wife Ethel, the woman he killed because she might have found him out. The prosecution suggested there were "significant actions" by which Christie showed both premeditation before the crime and desire to cover it up afterwards. First, eight days before the murder, he left his job with British Road Services, saying he was getting a job in Sheffield. That was untrue. Second, three days after the murder, he sold his wife's wedding ring. Third, he invented a whole series of untrue stories to account for his wife's absence from the neighbourhood. And fourth, he altered the date on a letter written by his wife on December 10th to December 15th, which was after her death, and sent it to her sister in Sheffield to give the impression that Mrs. Christie was still alive then.

The jury accepted the advice of Mr. Justice Finnemore in his summing-up, "The mere fact that a man acts like a monster, cruelly and wickedly, is not of itself evidence that he is insane," and found Christie guilty. He was hanged at Pentonville on Wednesday, July 15th, 1953.

The man who haunted the 10 Rillington Place trial – and has haunted the capital-punishment debate ever since – was Timothy John Evans. As Evans, who had lived on the top floor of the same house, went to the scaffold in 1950 on a charge of murdering his baby daughter Geraldine, two bodies lay in shallow graves in the garden, the bodies of Christie's first two victims.

The Christies and the Evanses became good friends and neighbours from Easter, 1948, but, according to

Christie, the Evanses had "terrific rows." The prosecution's case against Evans was that he strangled his wife in a fit of temper, and murdered his baby daughter at the same time. The Christies gave evidence against him at his trial, while all the time Evans protested his innocence. "I never done it, Mum, Christie done it," Evans said to his mother after his arrest.

Years later, after Evans was hanged, Christie was to confess that he himself had strangled Mrs. Evans while he was attempting to abort her of an unwanted pregnancy. "She said she would do anything if I would help her. I think she was referring to letting me be intimate with her. She brought the quilt from the front room and put it down in front of the fireplace. She lay on the quilt, fully dressed. I got on my knees but found I was not physically capable of having intercourse with her owing to the fibrosis in my back, and enteritis." When he killed her, he said, Evans (who was completely dominated by Christie) helped him carry the body downstairs. Later Christie, unknown to Evans, strangled little Geraldine.

In the summer of 1949 police discovered the bodies of the mother and child in the wash-house at 10 Rillington Place. At his trial Evans had ranged against him the persuasive John Christie, ex-special constable, whose cool, crisp evidence shone like a beacon against Evans's repeated contradictions and confusion. Even so, there were immediate doubts about the verdict. The forensic evidence that suggested that someone had attempted to have intercourse with Beryl Evans after she died was never properly addressed at the trial.

In 1966 Evans was granted a free pardon by the then Home Secretary, Roy Jenkins, following a committee of inquiry chaired by Mr. Justice Brabin. The judge said, "It is now impossible to establish the truth beyond doubt, but it is more probable than not that Evans did not kill his daughter."

Free pardons, of course, don't bring wrongly hanged men back to life. The case of Timothy Evans is evidence enough that despite all its sophistication, the law, like forensic science, is not infallible.

That forensic science might not be infallible was in no way better demonstrated than in the case of Norman Thorne, the Sussex poultry farmer who was hanged for killing his fiancée, dismembering her corpse and burying it in a chicken run. The girl, Elsie Cameron, used to leave her London home to spend weekends in what Thorne regarded as his home – a wooden shed set in the middle of his chickens, with just enough room in it for a trestle bed, a small table and a rickety chair. But his poverty belied his industry. Thorne worked hard, determined to make a go of the farm. He was a Sunday School teacher, a Band of Hope speaker, and both Elsie and Thorne were members of the Alliance for Chastity, and they planned to marry.

It was to be important to Thorne's defence after he was arrested that Elsie was a neurasthenic. She had lost one job after another because she was always having a crisis of nerves. Her first attack of depression was so bad that she had talked about committing suicide. So when her disappearance was reported to the police by her parents the case was not given much priority – certainly it was not filed under suspected murder. Elsie Cameron might never have been heard of again had not Thorne persistently insisted to reporters showing a mild interest in her disappearance that something sinister must have happened to her.

Until Elsie was found, he declared, his own position would always be one of compromise, for she had left home supposedly on a visit to him when she disappeared. "Something dreadful must have happened, I feel sure of it. Why should she commit suicide or run away when we were looking forward to a happy married life together? Why haven't I heard from her? Why haven't her parents heard anything? I can't understand why she left home on a Friday. She had written that I was to expect her as usual on Saturday at Groombridge station, but she wasn't there."

All this earnestness, though, received a sudden jolt when two men who lived in the village and a woman neighbour came forward to say they had seen a girl who looked like Elsie Cameron walking towards Thorne's hut at 5 p.m. on that Friday, December 5th, 1924. Thorne confidently assured the police that the witnesses must have been quite mistaken, but from that moment on there was a quickening of interest in the disappearance of Elsie Cameron. As Thorne joked that it was becoming common gossip that he had murdered her, Detective Chief Inspector Gillan of Scotland Yard arrived to investigate.

One of the first things the detective discovered was that Thorne had another girlfriend, Elizabeth Coldicott. Thorne had written to her, "I did not know that all this anxiety was coming or that we should begin to fall in love... Don't worry. I have a clear conscience, however things may look."

Thorne kept all his letters, including those he wrote to Elsie Cameron, and they revealed that her disappearance had come at a highly opportune time for him. They showed that she had been insisting on an early marriage because she was pregnant, and that Thorne had been using every subterfuge at his command to sidetrack her claims. They even showed that he had written to her confessing his affair with Elizabeth, to which Elsie replied,

"My own darling Norman – I've received your letter

this morning and you've absolutely broken my heart. I never thought you were capable of such deception. Had I gone off my head it would have been no excuse for you carrying on with another girl. You are engaged to me and I have the first claim. Your love for me (as you said you loved me) should have kept you true to me. It's a poor thing for a man to let himself go because his girl has her nerves bad (and the doctor told me when I went to be examined it was the way we had gone on that had made my nerves as they were, because knowing we were not married we had it on our minds that we might be found out)....You say you must have time to think, but whatever this girl expects of you, your duty is to marry me. Well, Norman, I expect you to marry me, and finish with the other girl as soon as possible. My baby must have a name, and another thing, I love you in spite of all. If anyone but yourself had told me another girl had been in your hut late at night I wouldn't have believed it.

With all my fondest love and kisses, forever your own loving Elsie."

This was a very damaging letter to Thorne. Gillan recognised that a clear motive for murder had been established, but the fact that Elsie Cameron was expecting to become a mother, and her lover was balking at marriage, was equally a reason for her to commit suicide.

Unable to extract a single incriminating admission from Thorne, Gillan ordered a party of policemen to start digging up the farm. By sheer luck they almost at once made a discovery that might have escaped them in a week's digging – Elsie's suitcase buried close to Thorne's hut. Among the things inside it was a baby's frock. Thorne was arrested.

As rain began to fall in a steady drizzle that evening Gillan called in digging reinforcements. The policemen worked ankle-deep in mud by the flaring light of oil torches and the dimmer illumination of lanterns. Soon one of the spades struck an obstacle. A moment or two later three bulky packages were lifted out of the damp earth. One was a battered old biscuit tin wrapped in rough sacking. The other two were heavy, limp bundles tied with string.

Inside the biscuit tin was a wrapped parcel, and inside the parcel was the head of a young girl, severed from the shoulders by someone who had cut down almost to the breast-bone, so that the neck was not mutilated – a method of dismemberment that was to be proved as being not without significance. The two other parcels contained other parts of the same body, and made up the complete corpse of Elsie Cameron.

After a whole day and an evening in the loneliness of his cell, Thorne sent for Gillan and made a belated admission that all the stories he had told since the girl's disappearance had been nothing but lies. But, he insisted, he did not kill Elsie. His story was that she walked in on him unexpectedly on the Friday evening and announced her intention of staying until he married her. After a long argument he told her had had to go out to keep an appointment with Elizabeth. Elsie reluctantly agreed.

"When I returned to the hut at about seven-thirty," Thorne's statement continued, "the dog came down to meet me. When I opened the hut door I saw Miss Cameron hanging from a beam by a piece of cord. I cut the cord and laid her on the bed. She was dead. I then put out the lights. She had her frock off and her hair was down. I went down to the workshop and got my hacksaw and some sacks and took them back to the hut. I tore off Miss Cameron's clothes and burned them in the fireplace. I then laid the sacks on the floor, put Miss Cameron (who was then naked) on the floor and sawed off the legs and the head by the glow of the fire. Next morning, just as it got light, I buried the sacks and a tin containing the remains in a chicken run."

The hanging story was not taken seriously at this stage, but when Sir Bernard Spilsbury was called in to do the post-mortem he was asked particularly to look for signs of hanging. He was to say that he found none – nor, incidentally, did he find any signs that Elsie was pregnant. He was emphatic that the girl had died from shock caused by severe injuries which had left extensive bruising on her body. There were two massive bruises on her head, one of which had reduced the tissues to pulp.

Gillan decided to put Thorne's story of a suicide to the test. He took with him a weight corresponding to the known weight of Elsie Cameron. In the hut the beam from which Thorne said he had cut down the girl was carefully examined. There was no dent in it. Gillan tied a length of cord to the beam, attached the weight to the cord, and let it drop. The pressure on the cord left a distinct groove in the soft wood. As he went about this reconstruction work Gillan also noticed significantly that the thick layer of dust on the top surface of the beam had not been disturbed in a very long time.

Six witnesses were marshalled by the defence to give medical evidence. Thorne told a reporter, "I know you think I'm going to be convicted, but I'm not. There is really only Spilsbury against me, and we'll soon knock down his evidence. I've a surprise in store that will startle people. You wait and see!"

Thorne's defence was so ingenious that it caused many notable logicians to argue that there was no legal proof he had committed murder. Even Sir Arthur Conan Doyle, creator of Sherlock Holmes, had his qualms. Strangely enough, the scene of the Elsie Cameron murder was not far from the country home of the great master of detective fiction.

Sir Arthur, however, made no personal first-hand investigation of the case. He formed conclusions simply from a study of the evidence at the trial. He summed up his unofficial opinion thus, "I am not quite easy about this case. In ninety-nine cases out of a hundred there are strong reasons for a conviction for murder. Personally, I am against capital punishment unless the murder has been definitely established. It is one thing to hang a man, but it is an impossible thing to bring him back to life. In the Thorne case, there does seem to be a faint doubt existing."

The trial of Norman Thorne is particularly memorable because despite his own terrible admissions, despite all the rest of the damning evidence piled up against him, Thorne put up one of the most remarkable fights for life ever seen in a British court of justice. It is even said that he planned his defence from the moment he started cutting up Elsie Cameron in his hut – deliberately removing the head so that the neck was intact. The reason he wanted to keep the neck intact was that he believed it showed marks indicative of hanging. So, carefully refraining from cutting straight across the throat, as almost any murderer would have done, he chose the harder task of cutting as close to the shoulders as possible to avoid lacerating the neck.

Throne kept his own counsel when Spilsbury gave evidence during the committal proceedings at the magistrates' court, evidence in which the famous pathologist said there were no signs of hanging on Elsie's neck. But back in prison he played what he regarded as his trump card. He sent for his lawyer and demanded that there be an exhumation of the girl's body.

"Spilsbury is wrong!" he declared with an air of triumph. "And we can prove it. I distinctly remember there were two red marks around Elsie's neck. If the body is exhumed you will see the clear proof that she hanged herself."

The Home Office granted an exhumation order, and Dr. Robert Brontë, an Irish pathologist, and his assistant, were appointed by the defence to carry out a second post-mortem on behalf of Thorne. The remains of Elsie Cameron had been buried in Willesden cemetery – now, four weeks later, they were dug up again. By this time the girl had been dead for three months, and her body had undergone considerable changes; even so, Brontë and his assistant managed to contradict Spilsbury's findings on a number of matters. Brontë was to tell the Assize Court at Lewes, where Thorne went on trial for his life on Thursday, March 4th, 1926, that the marks he found were consistent with an attempted hanging, cutting down before death, and then immediate death from shock. In various ways the pathologist was to be supported in his contentions by five other medical witnesses, while the prosecution rested their case entirely on Spilsbury, who told the court:

"I made a thorough search of the neck on January 17th [the date of the first post-mortem] because of the suggestion that the woman had died by hanging – not only externally but of the tissues under the skin. After I turned the skin back I cut across the creases, and in between fifteen and twenty such cuts I found no single area which suggested haemorrhage or which suggested crushing of the tissues, and no thickening or reddening of the skin itself resulting from pressure by a rope. There was no sign of any sort or kind of damage resulting from attempted hanging or actual hanging. It was therefore not necessary at that time to make any microscopic examination or to make slides. When the post-mortem was conducted by Dr. Brontë on February 24th the condition of the tissues was then such that no examination, microscopic or otherwise, would help. When the marks which I say were normal marks found on most women's necks were seen on February 24th by Dr. Brontë he made the remark which I took down at the time that they were 'the normal creases of the skin.' I have not the slightest doubt that they were... I took samples of the same parts of the skin of the right cheek and right side of the neck that Dr. Brontë had, and I made slides from these examples."

It is fair to say that Dr. Brontë denied that he had said at the post-mortem that the creases on Elsie's neck were natural or normal; they were grooves, he said, caused by the action of a thin rope or cord. He also claimed to have found extravasation (the breaking of blood vessels by violence or pressure). Death, in his view, was caused not by hanging but by shock from unsuccessful or interrupted attempt at self-strangulation, a way of death with which he was familiar. This suggested that Thorne must have cut down Emily before she was quite dead. The problem with Brontë's important contradictory evidence was that his methods, revealed under cross-examination, were seen to be rather less thorough than Spilsbury's. The specimen slides made for the defence were not all made by Brontë himself, and some of them revealed only decomposition. Against that it had to be seen that Spilsbury had made no slides at the first post-mortem, arguing that the causes of the shock that brought on death were so obvious that microscopic investigation simply wasn't necessary.

Spilsbury stuck to his guns. So insistent was he that he went on to say that he found signs to rebut the defence suggestion, which were "injuries on the head, face, elbow, legs, and feet, which together were amply sufficient to account for death from shock, and death which must have occurred very shortly after those injuries were inflicted. I found nothing else at all to

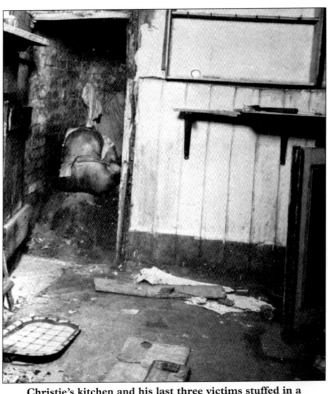

Christie's kitchen and his last three victims stuffed in a cupboard. Below, after removal of each of the bodies

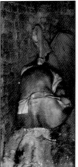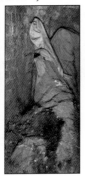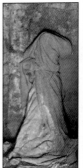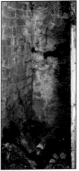

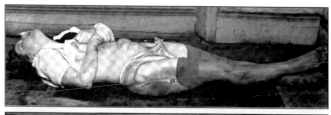

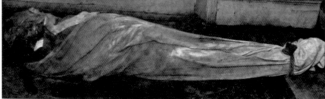

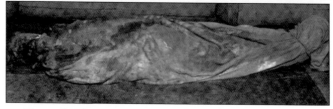

Above, the three victims after removal from the cupboard.
Below, John Christie and his wife. Her body (right) was found
beneath the floorboards

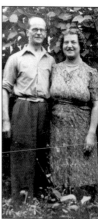

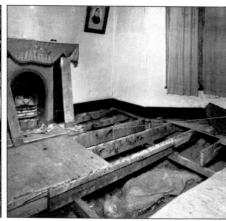

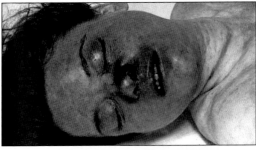

Left and below, Christie's last victim, showing ligature marks around her neck

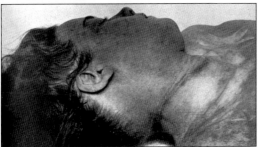

See chapter 6

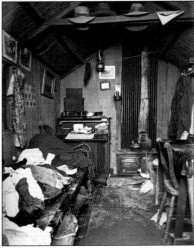

Inside Norman Thorne's hut. Note the beam. It was from another of these that Thorne claimed Elsie had hanged herself

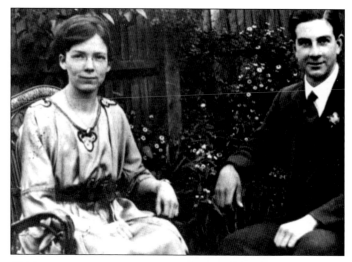

Chicken farmer Norman Thorne and his girl friend Elsie Cameron

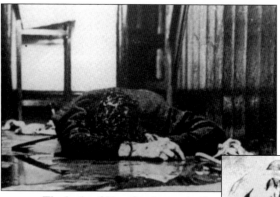

The body of Mrs. Sandeman in the hallway of The Crag.
Right, the wounds of a victim who committed suicide using an axe

See chapter 8

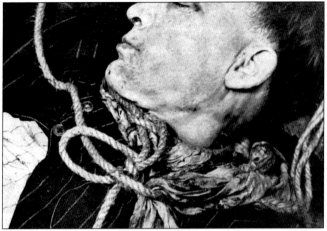

John Mudie as he was found in a shallow grave in a Surrey chalkpit
See chapter 9

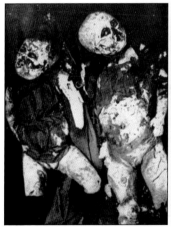

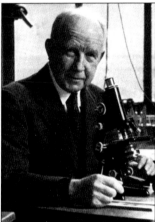

Above, the bodies of the
children found in the
Hopetoun Quarry. Top right,
Sir Sydney Smith, and right,
an arm and a leg from the
brothers which are still used
at Edinburgh University as
examples of adipocere

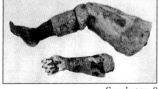

See chapter 9

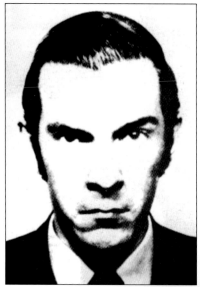

Poison, the silent killer. Graham Young (left) had a preference for thallium, while Louisa Merrifield (below) used phosphorus

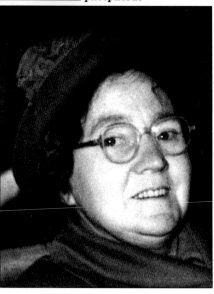

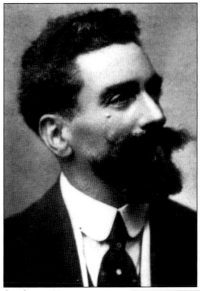

Jean-Pierre Vaquier had purchased the strychnine in London

See chapter 11

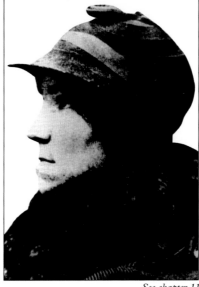

Charlotte Bryant. The poison she chose was arsenic

See chapter 11

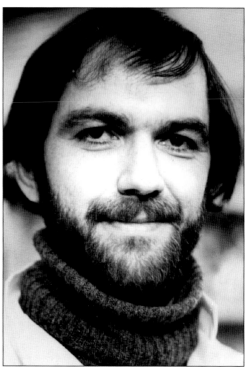

The discovery that made DNA a method of positive identification was made by Professor Alec Jeffreys (left) in 1984

See chapter 12

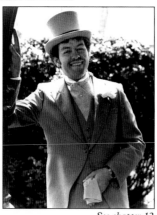

Colin Pitchfork was the first murderer in the world to be caught by DNA fingerprinting

See chapter 12

account for death." When a rope was produced in court he studied it and said that such a rope would immediately make a mark on the neck; "there was no such mark."

Mr. Justice Finlay, who presided at the trial, sanctioned a conference between the contending experts in the hope that they would arrive at some agreement. The doctors studied their slides and debated their differences in private, but both sides refused to budge an inch. They were utterly at variance over their conclusions. The only thing on which they could agree was that Elsie did not die from hanging. The defence doctors insisted on Thorne's behalf that it was conceivable the girl had died from shock while in the act of attempting suicide by hanging herself.

It can be argued on behalf of Thorne that the unusual way in which he decapitated the corpse is corroborative of the hanging story – it showed he realised the necessity of preserving the evidence of his innocence. It can be just as strongly argued that he had already worked out the hanging story at the time of dismemberment, that the unusual decapitation was all part of his master plan.

But there is much that tells against him. Evidently he seemed to be in no state of panic, so why did he have to dismember the corpse? If he came back to his hut and saw Elsie dead from hanging – or almost dead, as the forensic evidence indicated – why did he not simply call the police? Then there was the indisputable fact that Elsie died after a struggle. Her glasses were found broken in her suitcase, and the locket she was wearing was torn from its chain.

Thorne was nothing if not cunning. He was a student of criminal cases. A book on pathology and newspaper clippings of two sensational murder cases were discovered in his hut. In both these cases the body of the victim had been dismembered. Thorne had gone to great pains to avoid making the mistakes that had brought those criminals to justice.

Why then had he been so anxious to preserve the neck if there had been no hanging or attempted hanging? The answer surely is that he knew Elsie had suicidal tendencies. So when her body was stretched out on the floor of his hut he simulated a death by hanging by putting a cord around her neck and pulling on it with all his might. He would not have known that post-mortem marks do not remain like those made during life – that strangulation after death does not leave the traces that are left by strangulation that is the cause of death.

Thorne remained icily calm throughout his trial. He gave his evidence with all the self-assurance in the world, but a man who tells a story of dismembering his sweetheart's body and recites it with no more show of emotion than if he had been addressing one of his Sunday school classes makes a bad impression on the jury. They found him guilty of murder. He staggered visibly under the unexpected blow of the death sentence. A deathly pallor settled over his face when the black cap was draped over Mr Justice Finlay's wig.

In the condemned cell, with his last hope of reprieve gone, Thorne read his Bible diligently, his piety knowing no bounds.

"The world seems bright and beautiful," he wrote in his farewell letter to his parents, "but how much better must be the Kingdom of Heaven to a believer! Try to grasp the real meaning of this and your sorrow will fade away as mine has in the shadow of darkness. A flash and all is finished, no not finished, but just starting, and I shall wait for you just as others are waiting for me."

Thorne was hanged at Wandsworth Prison on Wednesday, April 22nd, 1925, on what would have been Elsie Cameron's 25th birthday. A number carved on a flagstone in the prison cemetery marks his simple grave.

Although Spilsbury effectively demolished Thorne's claim that Elsie had committed suicide, nothing can be taken absolutely for granted when a decision has to be made between suicide and murder. In a case in which suicide would seem to have been entirely ruled out, it was claimed by the defence that the victim had actually killed herself and had not been murdered. It happened in October, 1942, when a 16-year-old nursemaid, Sheila Ferguson, was accused of murdering her employer Mrs. Eva Sandeman, aged 37, with an axe. Mrs. Sandeman had been found lying in a pool of blood at her rented house, The Crag, overlooking the beach in the Cornish village of Seaton. Axe murderers are a rarity; women axe murderers are rarer still since the days of the legendary Lizzie Borden. But Sheila's astonishing defence was that Mrs. Sandeman committed suicide – by killing herself with the axe.

The nursemaid had been seen hurrying away from The Crag with the Sandemans' three children, all of whom were weeping. She had a cut hand. Police called to the house thought Mrs. Sandeman had been attacked by a maniac.

Sheila Ferguson claimed that she was first attacked by Mrs. Sandeman, who also attacked the children. She could give no reason for her employer's behaviour. She said that after attacking her, Mrs. Sandeman turned the axe on herself, a story that did not account for the fact that some of the wounds were inflicted after death. As far as the nursemaid was concerned, when she left the house with the children Mrs. Sandeman was lying in the hall on her back with two self-inflicted wounds on her face.

According to Sheila, Mrs. Sandeman "raised the hatchet and struck herself a blow on the forehead.

Then a second time she struck herself about the nostrils or right eye. She then collapsed on her back, with blood covering her face and most of her hair."

Impossible? Not quite, because there have been self-inflicted deaths using an axe. The suicide usually aims the axe against the forehead and crown of the head. The first blows are light, but get harder as the suicide uses more and more force.

The jury refused to believe, though, that this happened in the Cornish killing. They found Sheila Ferguson not guilty of murder but guilty of manslaughter. She was sentenced to be detained for five years, and died shortly after completing the sentence.

A murderer who did use an axe to kill, not once but twice, was caught in 1992 by the single forensic clue he left on his discarded murder weapon.

His first victim was 75-year-old Farmer Fred Maltby, who lived alone in his farmhouse outside Lincoln. Police found four deep gashes in Maltby's head, one of which had fractured his skull. There was no murder weapon, no motive and no suspect. There was, though, one slender clue. After killing Maltby the murderer put the weapon down on the settee, leaving the impression of a full-sized axe-head outlined in his victim's blood. He probably searched the house for money, then picked up the axe and walked off with it. The bloody print revealed only that the axe was square at one end and tapered at the other. The only other thing that could be deduced was that the victim must have known his killer and let him in.

With no other clues to follow, the investigation was soon floundering, and remained so until four months later when, in January, 1992, bookmaker Joe Rylatt, 62, was found battered to death in his Lincoln betting shop. His safe door hung open and nearly £3,000 was missing.

Detectives investigating the murder discovered that Rylatt was something of a small-time moneylender. In his diary they found a list of the names of people who had borrowed money from him. Each name was checked out, but none of them could be linked to the murder.

Detective Superintendent Stuart Clifton, who was still leading the investigation into the killing of Fred Maltby, was intrigued by the wounds in Joe Rylatt's head – they were identical to those on Maltby. He examined them with a microscope and spotted tiny fragments of paint deep in the gashes. Reasoning that they must have come from the axe head, he sent them for analysis. All that this revealed was that the paint contained a lot of zinc, but it could not be identified.

Clifton went on TV to appeal for anyone finding an axe to take it to their local police station and almost at once four young boys came up with an axe which they had found on an island in the middle of a local boating pond. Blood traces on the axe-head were examined and were revealed to have come from Joe Rylatt. Knowing that this was the murder weapon, Clifton scraped more paint from the axe-head and sent it to the British Paint Research Foundation.

The Foundation's report was to give Clifton his first big lead. The paint, it said, contained traces of a rare binding agent, Epoxyester D4, and it was made only in Essen, in Germany. The zinc it contained was not new, but had been reconstituted.

Clifton went to Essen, where the manufacturers of Epoxyester D4 gave him a list of the factories which bought their binding agent, outlets which were spread all over northern Europe. Painstakingly, working at it for weeks on end, he phoned them all, asking if they used a binding agent in their paint which contained reconstituted zinc, and if so, did they export it to England. At last his industry paid off. A Dutch factory told him that they not only made that type of paint, but they had sold it to only one outlet in England via an agency in Wolverhampton.

At Clifton's request the agency then went through their records, checking the customers they had supplied with the paint. One of them, a London firm of builder's merchants, had bought 36 cans. They still had 12 cans: the rest had been sold to a firm next door called Specialist Heat Exchangers.

Clifton studied a list of the staff who worked for Specialist Heat Exchanges. One of the names was Denis Granville Smalley, employed as a welder. Clifton knew the name from memory – Smalley was on the list of people who had borrowed money from Joe Rylatt found in the bookmaker's diary.

Now detectives began a detailed trawling through the life of Denis Smalley. They checked his alibi; he had said he had been baby-sitting at home while his wife was at work on the day that Joe Rylatt was killed. They discovered that a neighbour, incensed at the way she thought Smalley was neglecting his children, had kept a diary of his comings and goings. On the night Joe Rylatt was murdered she recorded that Smalley left his house for nearly two hours – the same two hours during which the bookmaker was killed. Next they checked his financial situation to find out what caused him to borrow money from the bookmaker. They found he had owed nearly £18,000 before Joe Rylatt was killed, and that after the murder he was clearing some of his debts. Then they checked with the relatives of Farmer Maltby to see if they knew of Smalley.

"Did you ever hear of a man named Denis Smalley?" they asked Maltby's sister.

"Why, yes," she replied. "Fred hired him as a part-time hand."

"But you told us before that he never hired anyone."

"I thought you meant full-time employees," replied the sister. "He never hired full-time employees. Only part-time men. Smalley worked part-time for him once."

Armed with all this evidence, which had begun with only the axe itself, Clifton arrested Denis Smalley. Detectives who searched the welder's house found a can of priming paint in his garage. Part of its contents were Epoxyester D4 and reconstituted zinc. Although Smalley had used the grey primer to paint the axe-head after he killed Fred Maltby, the axe still bore traces of blood which was proved to have come from Joe Rylatt.

Denis Smalley, 48, was tried at Lincoln Crown Court in July, 1994. Among the witnesses was Stephen Jones, professor of forensic medicine at Nottingham University, who said that axe-murders were so rare he had come across only two other such fatal attacks in 23 years of being called to the scene of hundreds of killings.

"The weapon in this case was a heavy one with a fairly sharp blade," he said. "The edges were not absolutely clear cut – they were a little bit on the ragged side." The injuries to both victims bore similar characteristics, and were made with the same weapon.

Found guilty of both murders, Denis Smalley was given two life terms of life imprisonment. The judge, Mr. Justice Holland, had words of praise for super-sleuth Stuart Clifton, congratulating him on the "remarkable skill and determination" he had shown throughout the investigation.

9

HANGING AND DROWNING

*After the killer was hanged, his body was rendered
down to its skeleton and then wired up for the
benefit of future forensic scientists*

Although all the best evidence is against it, let us
suppose for a moment that Elsie Cameron did try
to hang herself that night in Thorne's hut while he was
out with another girl friend. If a pathologist had been
almost immediately summoned – as would have been
the case if Thorne had called the police – he would
have found an unusually pale face and dilated pupils.
The lips and tongue would have been bluish, a
discoloration caused by deoxygenated blood. The
ligature line would depend on the type of noose used,
but the mark of the ligature would have most likely
followed the line of the lower jaw before proceeding up
behind the ear, pulled in that direction by the weight
of the body. The cause of death would have been
asphyxia (literally, lack of oxygen), so the brain would
be congested, and there might have been bleeding in
the trachea and larynx. Additionally, the thyroid
cartilage might have been broken, and the hyoid bone
fractured. It does not need a pathologist to explain
that Thorne would have had an exceedingly difficult
task to simulate a hanging death, and had he not cut
up his fiancée's body the pathologist would have
immediately started to look for injuries which might
provide clues as to the real cause of death.

Hanging is a common form of suicide, and one that is comparatively easily effected. But cases exist of extraordinary attempts by suicides to pass off their deaths as murders. One such happened at the Ritz Hotel in London in 1953, when a man and a woman were found dead in a double room. Police were at first convinced that it was a double murder. The woman lay on the floor with her throat cut. The man was suspended from the top frame of the bed by a cord around his neck, and part of his body weight was supported by a pillow on the floor. A scarf had been placed between the cord and the neck, and a sock was stuffed into his mouth.

In the bathroom there were bloodstains on the floor and the mirror, and a trail of bloodstains led to the bed. When the scarf was removed from the man's neck a pathologist discovered slight wounds made by a razor. It was deduced that the man had killed the woman by cutting her throat with a razor and had then tried unsuccessfully to cut his own throat in the bathroom. After that he stuffed a sock into his mouth, put a scarf around his neck to make the ligature more comfortable, and then hanged himself by the cord, letting himself down gently on the pillow.

In another case the victim had tied his wrists together, and then with remarkable agility succeeded in passing his legs and his body between his arms, so that his hands were then tied together over his backside. Stepping on a chair he passed his head through a noose and hanged himself. Again, police called to the scene were at first convinced that it must be murder.

But murder it certainly was, detectives decided, when they were called to a heavily waterlogged chalkpit near Woldingham, Surrey, on a Sunday morning in November, 1946, to view the corpse of a man with a noose around his neck who was lying in a shallow grave. The grave in fact was more of a trench that had been dug some time previously – it hadn't been especially made for the corpse. It was half-filled with fresh earth, which suggested that someone had begun to bury the body and had been interrupted. The clothes were pulled up over the shoulders, and the shoes were clean and dry – all indicators that the body must have been dragged to the chalkpit.

The noose around the neck was puzzling. Murder by hanging? This is distinctly unusual. Hanging is very much the choice of suicides, but someone who has hanged himself can't then drag his body to a shallow trench, lie down in it and die. Hypostasis and rigor mortis revealed that the body must have arrived in its grave at the time of death or soon after it. The post-mortem cause of death was given as asphyxia. The rope around the neck had left a distinct mark, but the shape of the mark was not that of a ligature. It rose to a point under the ear on the left side, producing the inverted V that is characteristic of hanging as the head lolls over to the other side. There was a green cloth between the rope and the neck, the sort of barrier used by suicides to soften the effect of the ligature on the skin. There were some bruises and abrasions too, but not sufficient to have been caused by the victim's struggles while being hanged against his will.

Forensic pathologist Dr. Eric Gardner decided that the man had been dead for forty-eight hours, and that in some way his body must have been suspended. There was no place above or around the chalkpit where this could have happened, so it must have occurred somewhere else, and the body been brought to the chalkpit.

The corpse was that of John Mudie, aged 35, a barman at the Reigate Hill Hotel, ten miles away; he was identified from information found in his pockets. He was last seen three days previously. What was to prove an excellent clue was provided when two men reported having seen a suspicious character in the chalkpit. They watched him until he noticed them, whereupon he jumped into a small car and drove off at speed. The witnesses took the car's registration number, which included the figures 101.

Letters on John Mudie tied him to a Mrs. Byron Brook, who lodged in the same Wimbledon house where Mudie had lived. Mrs. Brook was the director of a property company owned by a Thomas Ley, of Beaufort Gardens, Kensington, and apparently knowing that they were so to speak neighbours, Ley had sent some letters to Mudie for Mrs. Brook, asking him to pass them on. The letters contained cheques, and Mudie had passed them to Mrs. Brook's daughter. The cheques had not reached Mrs. Brook, causing Ley to suggest that Mudie must have stolen them.

Detectives investigating these leads concentrated their attention on Thomas Ley. He was a former Minister of Justice in New South Wales, and was in his sixties. He had been having an affair with Mrs. Brook, and although she had met John Mudie only once in their lodging-house, Ley had conceived the obsessive idea that Mudie was having an affair with her. Deciding that Ley must somehow be involved in the death of Mudie, Surrey police called in Scotland Yard.

Dr. Gardner told the Yard's Detective Chief Inspector Arthur Philpott that in his view the injuries on Mudie's body suggested he had been beaten up. This was hardly likely to have been done by Ley, so there must have been an accomplice. Philpott surmised that Ley might have hired someone to give Mudie a beating but not to kill him, and it had all gone wrong. A story was fed to the newspapers, and as a result a former professional boxer, John Buckingham, went to the police and confessed that

Ley had paid him £200 to kidnap Mudie, who according to Ley was blackmailing a woman friend of his. Buckingham named his accomplice in the kidnapping as Lawrence Smith, a carpenter who had worked on Ley's house.

So what had happened to the unfortunate John Mudie? Buckingham claimed that he and Smith took the barman to Ley's house, pushed him into a room and left him there. There was no struggle. Smith, interviewed separately, told a different story. He said he held Mudie from in front, pinioning his arms downwards and standing in front of him, while Buckingham threw a rug over him from behind. They wound a rope around the blanket, then jumped Mudie out of the room into another room. During this procedure Mudie fell forward with Buckingham on top of him. They picked him up and set him down in a swivel chair. Smith then found a rag to gag Mudie, and Buckingham pulled the rug up from Mudie's face and tied the gag around his mouth. (The gag was the same piece of cloth found on Mudie's body between the cord and his neck.) When they left, leaving Mudie in the swivel chair, the barman was conscious. Shown Smith's statement, Buckingham agreed that he had thrown a rug over Mudie's head, and that he had jumped him out of the room, but he denied that Mudie had fallen, or that he had been gagged.

Evidently there was some kind of a fracas when Mudie was brought to Ley's house, sufficient perhaps to support Dr. Gardner's view of a beating up, the effects of which would have been softened by the rug. The involvement of the three men was further confirmed when it was discovered that Smith had hired a small Ford car just before the murder, and that its registration number was 101. One of the witnesses who had seen a man behaving suspiciously at the chalkpit the day before the murder identified

Lawrence Smith as that man, which suggested that Smith had played a bigger part in the proceedings than he had admitted. There was still no one prepared to say that Mudie was hoisted up, an action which caused his death.

To bolster their case the prosecution allowed Buckingham to turn King's evidence, and Ley and Smith were put on trial for murder. The trial was unusual because Dr. Keith Simpson, the Home Office pathologist who had monitored the case, appeared as a witness for the defence – a situation which grew out of Simpson's unease about the case. Later he was to write, "I found no reason to think Mudie had suffered any injury to the brain or stomach and intestine... I did not like the idea of trying to fit medical observations to the details of a statement." Another surprise defence witness was a man named Robert Cruikshank, a friend of Ley's who had a criminal record. He said he went to Ley's house and found a man there trussed up in a chair. Cruikshank pulled at the rope in a panic – now he wondered if he had possibly killed the man by accident. Simpson, asked if this were possible, said anyone who had lifted the rope and held it for two or three minutes could have killed Mudie.

In the witness box Dr. Gardner said Mudie could have been injured only in falling, and posed the probability of a "contre-coup" – forensic parlance for a blow on the back of the head which crushes the front of the brain. As far as the rope marks on the neck were concerned "there was an indication of some tension upwards, some form of suspension, but he had not been hanged in the ordinary sense of the word." Dr. Simpson's view was that Mudie had been "drawn and lifted – it was the lifting that did it." But accident, suicide or murder, he could not say.

What actually happened to John Mudie that day in

Kensington will never be known, but one thing is for sure – the full story was not revealed at the trial. Despite the disputed medical evidence, though, there was plenty of other evidence against the two prisoners, and Ley and Smith were both found guilty and sentenced to death. After the sentencing Ley was found insane by a Medical Board and died a few months later in Broadmoor. Smith missed the hangman – his sentence was commuted to life imprisonment.

Judicial hanging, abolished in the UK in 1965, began in Anglo-Saxon times and continued to be the punishment employed for many crimes until the nineteenth century, when the penal code was rewritten by Sir Robert Peel. For hundreds of years hanging for the offence of treason was refined by cutting down the victim before he choked to death, cutting out his bowels while he was still just about alive, burning them in front of him, then cutting him into four pieces which were stuck on poles and exhibited as a warning to others. Even after the abolition of hanging, drawing and quartering, judicial hanging continued to be no more than slow strangulation. When John Lomas was hanged at Chester Castle for killing his girlfriend's husband in 1812 hanging was a melodramatic affair. On the morning of August 24, the execution day, the prison's deputy governor took Lomas around the jail to say his farewells to everyone. He was then led to the scaffold, fitted up over the main door of the castle so that the crowd could look up from the road below. Lomas died gallantly, twitching on the end of the rope for several minutes. His body was rendered down to its skeleton, which was then sent to London, where it was wired up for the benefit of future forensic scientists.

Just before dawn on December that same year Edith Morrey, Lomas's girlfriend who had been implicated in the murder of her husband, gave birth in prison to a boy who was named Thomas Morrey. By the law of the day she could be hanged one month after the birth. In fact the execution was delayed until April 23rd. At 8 a.m., after saying her farewells, she was put in a cart and driven along a ninety-yard stretch of road lined with sightseers to the gallows. As the wheels rolled over the cobbles church bells tolled mournfully. Undeterred by the heavy sky and sharp easterly wind, a crowd of 10,000 had arrived outside Chester prison to watch her die.

Much of the crowd's noise and rowdyism was provoked by the hangman. Sammy Burrows habitually carried out preparations with a perky insolence that made him a darling of the masses, but which more sensitive souls found distasteful. He began his routine by balancing on a stool and trying to lasso the crossbar. When these antics were over Edith submitted to the tying. First her forearms were pinioned in front, hands lashed together as if clasped in prayer. This was meant to stop her shifting the noose once it had been put in position with the knot behind her left ear. The next stage was a blush-saving relic of pre-drop days, when women on the scaffold were pushed off a ladder leaning against the upright. For this Burrows criss-crossed another length of cord around Edith's skirt from knees to ankles. This was nevertheless done to the accompaniment of ribald comments, before the halter was arranged.

After the chaplain had intoned Burrows placed Edith on the trap-door, and tucked a handkerchief between her hands to be released as a signal when she was ready. Then he covered her face with a square of white material. This last act was not for her sake but to protect the sensibilities of those standing by. When the trap-door fell, head and shoulders would still be visible. The expression of anyone whose windpipe has been suddenly and violently constricted was known to be a very ugly sight.

Burrows went below and shot the bolt; the crowd saw a parcelled-up piece of humanity plunge downwards. Pulled up short, it started jerking. A reporter from the *Chester Chronicle* timed the spasms; they went on, he wrote, for two and a half minutes.

The *Chester Chronicle* had been told that the dissection of Edith's corpse would be a token affair only – and the vindictive editor couldn't believe it. If Lomas had been so thoroughly processed that only his skeleton was left, then the same treatment should be suffered by "the wretched woman who instigated him to be a principal in the horrid crime." Somehow a journalist gained admission to the dissection, which was systematically reported in a blow-by-blow account in the *Chester Chronicle* that left nothing to the imagination in this unpleasant side of not-so-Old England.

According to the newspaper, the day after the execution Dr. James Titley made an incision in the throat of the corpse – just below a discoloured seam of scar tissue around the wound caused by Edith's attempt to cut her own throat immediately before her arrest – along the line of the sternum. His next strokes laid bare the thoracic cavity. After the breast bone itself and part of the rib cage had been sawn through and lifted out, a perfect view was obtained of the heart, lungs, and cardiovascular system. Finally, using a broad-bladed scalpel and forceps, Titley extended the original incision downwards, opening up the abdominal cavity and exposing the viscera, "et cetera." The "et cetera" apparently sufficed for what the *Chester Chronicle* declined to name. Titley then excised the heart, which was sealed in a jar of alcohol.

The corpse was stitched up again and put on show to the public, who paid a few pence per head to stand in line and gawk at it. Then it was whisked away, probably to relatives. The newspaper's view of that was expressed unequivocally: "We have no doubt that if application was made for the body, it was delivered up to those who had more relative claims upon it and that humanity alone sanctioned the concession."

A postscript to the story which must have had nineteenth-century moralists clucking in unison was that little Thomas Morrey, born in prison four months before his mother's execution, grew up at odds with the law. For stealing a few things, including two live hens and a pair of socks, he was transported to Australia for seven years. He was last heard of in a penal colony in Hobart, Tasmania, in 1834.

Even in our own century judicial hanging, abolished in the UK in 1965, was steeped in ritual from the moment the judge donned the black cap until the victim dropped through the scaffold trap-door. Perhaps death didn't even end there. The renowned forensic pathologist Sir Sydney Smith never forgot the first execution he attended in his official capacity. He wrote in his autobiography, "Death, said the prison doctor, was instantaneous, but when I felt the pulse of the executed man, still feebly beating, I wondered at the calm certainty with which my medical colleague pronounced his verdict." In judicial hanging the upper cervical vertebrae – the neck – are dislocated and the spinal cord severed, but when does the victim actually die? Undoubtedly the heart continues to beat for a second or two after death, so can there still be consciousness after the neck is broken? Sydney Smith retells the story, which he thinks may be apocryphal, of Sir Everard Digby, executed for his role in the Guy Fawkes plot to blow up Parliament. The headsman took out Digby's heart and showed it to the audience, proclaiming, "This is the heart of a traitor." Some were to declare afterwards that the head distinctly replied, "Thou liest."

Like hanging, drowning is not chosen by many murderers as their method of killing, but drowned bodies are an all too familiar sight on the pathologist's examination table. One of the more obvious external signs of drowning when the body is seen soon after death is the appearance of a watery mucous froth around the nostrils and lips. The skin is also pale and wrinkled, and in cold water "goose-pimpled." But the absence of these appearances would not prove that the victim had not been drowned, for if the body had been in the water for some time, or exposed to air for a long time before examination, there may be other changes, and there may no longer be mucus and froth.

Another external sign of drowning is cadaveric spasm – the discovery of some object like a piece of wood or weeds from the bank of a river, locked in the victim's clenched hand. This would have been grabbed during the struggle for life and not released in death.

The process of drowning causes fluid to be sucked into the lungs, from where a good deal of it will enter the bloodstream. So internally one way of identifying a drowning case is by the presence of diatoms in the blood or in the bone marrow. Diatoms are microscopic algae found in ponds, rivers, and seas; their silica shells are resistant to acids. At the post-mortem the pathologist takes a piece of tissue from the victim and dissolves it in acid. If there are any diatoms they will remain, and can be seen under the microscope, indicating that because they could only have got into the victim by way of the bloodstream the victim must have been alive in the water. Very few or no diatoms would indicate that death took place before the victim went into the water.

Sometimes the head of a drowned person is discoloured from putrefaction when the rest of the body seems unchanged – this is because the head of a submerged body floats lower than the rest of the body, causing blood to gravitate to the head and neck, encouraging bacterial growth. When a body has been in water for several days the palms of the hands and the soles of the feet become thick and white. The body is sodden, so that bruises and other marks of violence made before death are not apparent until water has evaporated from the skin.

A drowned body eventually rises to the surface because of gaseous putrefaction. The time this takes depends mostly on the temperature of the water. In summer it will usually rise after two or three days – in winter it may take as long as six weeks if the water is cold. After a fortnight of immersion the skin of the fingers becomes detached, and the hair can be wiped away. After several months the muscles become soft and discoloured, and the fatty parts may be converted into adipocere. Finally the soft parts of the body are washed away, leaving the skeleton. In a case of drowning, therefore, the shorter the time the body has been immersed the more information the forensic scientist is likely to retrieve from it.

In the double murder known as the Thames Towpath case the body of Christine Reed, 18, was discovered in the Thames five days after she had been beaten with an axe, stabbed and thrown into the river. Almost a week earlier police had found the body of another girl, Barbara Songhurst, 16, who in addition to having been beaten and stabbed, had also been raped. If Christine too had been raped the murders would be identical, and the manhunt would be for a sex killer. Forensic pathologists who examined Christine's body knew that in warm weather (this was midsummer, 1953) a thick covering of algae may form over the exposed parts of an immersed body. This coat of algae, if formed rapidly enough, will give protection to the body from attacks by small animals, and will seal up the body's orifices. In Christine's case the vagina had been completely sealed by the algae, and the vaginal contents were therefore uncontaminated. These contents were examined under a microscope, and spermatozoa were immediately recognisable. The forensic experts were able to conclude that Christine was raped, and not quite so conclusively they considered that she was also raped after she died.

In the face of formidable evidence against him, the towpath killer, Alfred Whiteway, a 22-year-old builder's labourer with no previous history of violence, confessed, then retracted the confession. He was tried at the Old Bailey in October, 1953, found guilty, and hanged at Wandsworth Prison on December 22nd the same year.

Forensic pathologists have a library of knowledge of what happens to a drowned body. They know that the lungs of a victim are pale and distended, completely filling the chest cavity, and they remain wet – touch them with a finger and the impression remains. The throat and bronchi are filled with a watery mucous froth, tinged sometimes with blood, as a result of the last desperate efforts to breathe. The stomach may also contain water, swallowed during the pre-death struggle. The blood is dark in colour, which is caused by the absorption of all available oxygen and consequent reduction of the haemoglobin.

Generally bodies decompose more slowly in water than out of it, since for most of the year water temperature remains below atmospheric temperature. When the water temperature is continuously below 40-45 degrees Fahrenheit a body may show very little decomposition after several weeks' immersion. At 50-70 degrees Fahrenheit it may start decomposing after four days. In the tropics it may begin decomposition within 24 hours.

In the early part of the twentieth century an extraordinary case of body immersion and decomposition occurred, where the forensic findings led to the arrest and execution of a brutally callous killer. It began when two young ploughmen, Peter Aitken and Jack Summers, went for a walk on a Sunday morning. They had been strolling through the fields and woods around Winchburgh, near Stirling, when they came to a disued quarry at Hopetoun. Newly topped up with summer rain, the quarry was 100 yards long, 40 yards across and in places 40 feet deep. It wasn't a place that was much frequented by the local working folk, who didn't pass their Sundays going for walks. But Aitken was showing Summers, who was new to the district, something of the countryside, so there was a method in their excursion.

As the quarry waters came in sight Summers said, "Look over there. Someone's thrown an old scarecrow into the water."

The two men advanced cautiously, instinctively aware that something might be wrong, for Hopetoun Quarry didn't seem the kind of place that anyone would want to throw a scarecrow. As they drew near Aitken said quietly, "It isn't a scarecrow. It looks more like a human body to me."

A yard or two more and it was clear that Aitken was right. The scarecrow was a body – or rather two small bodies lashed together. The two men waded into the water and lowered a tree branch under the cord holding the two little forms, in order to pull them into the bank. But the branch broke, and so too did the cord.

"We'd better fetch the police," Aitken said.

That afternoon in June, 1913, the police took the two bodies to the Linlithgow mortuary, where forensic pathologist Sydney Smith and Professor Harvey Littlejohn, head of forensic medicine at Edinburgh University, arrived to examine them. The first thing they noticed was that despite their intensive state of decomposition the bodies were still clothed. Forensic scientists are like detectives in that they are trained to take everything into account – frequently the artefacts on or around a body can tell at least as much as the state of the body itself. The clothes were cheap, and both boys were dressed exactly alike, suggesting that they might be brothers. Although the clothes fell apart at a touch because of their long immersion in water, Smith was able to identify a stamp on one of the small shirts. It was the mark of the Dysart workhouse in Fife.

Unclothed, the two bodies presented an unusual sight. As a result of a long immersion they had become virtually transformed into adipocere. This, as we have seen, is the chemo-physical change that occurs when a body is buried in damp ground or is left for a long time in water. Human fat, normally semi-fluid, is slowly converted to a fat which is quite firm, like suet – adipocere. Once a body reaches an adipocerous condition it cannot return to its original state. In the case of the two bodies pulled from Hopetoun Quarry the transformation was complete except for the feet, which were protected from the action of water on the tissues by their boots.

There was no doubt that they were human, so the next question was their sex. Although the adipocere had preserved the shape of the bodies, the sex was far from clear. Smith thought that one looked more like a girl than a boy, but when he cut into the groin he found male glandular structures. In fact both bodies were those of boys.

How long had they been in the water? Smith decided it was probably somewhere between 18 months and two years. That meant they must have been put there the year before last – in 1911.

There is no better measure for deciding the age of a dead child in decomposition than its teeth, for there are regular changes to teeth in human beings almost from birth until adulthood. The bigger boy had cut his first permanent molars, which put him around the age of six. His central incisors were also fully cut; usually these erupt about the age of seven. The lateral incisors, which usually erupt at the age of eight, were being formed. All the other teeth were milk teeth. Taking all this into account, and after examining the growing ends of the boy's long bones, Smith decided he must have been about seven years old when he died. The smaller boy had none of his permanent teeth but all of his milk teeth, as would be the case of a child aged between two and six. The first permanent molars had almost appeared, suggesting, together with the condition of the bones, that his age was between three and four.

Then by a remarkable piece of forensic work Smith was able to announce exactly what the two boys had eaten for their last meal, and how long after they had eaten it that they died. This was because astonishingly the stomach contents of both of them had been preserved intact by the extensive adipocere formation. What Smith found was some thick material that included undigested and easily recognisable vegetable matter, such as barley, potatoes, turnips, leeks and whole green peas. These, he pointed out, were the traditional ingredients for Scotch broth, and the undigested state of the matter suggested that the meal had not been eaten more than an hour before they died. This in turn suggested that the children lived locally.

Smith and Littlejohn set out to walk to Hopetoun Quarry themselves, going over the last tracks on earth taken by the two little boys. They reasoned that the boys may have walked to the quarry with their killer, since no wheeled vehicle could have negotiated the rough country. He must have murdered them by the water's edge – Smith was unable to say how – tied the bodies together, and thrown them into the water. And because of the loneliness of the spot, there they stayed for what was subsequently deduced as twenty months.

With so much forensic evidence to go on, the police searched through their files for reports of children reported missing during the previous two years. They discovered that two brothers, one aged almost seven and the other aged four, had unaccountably disappeared in November, 1911.

Their father, Patrick Higgins, was an Irishman who had once served in the Indian Army; now he was known to be a consummate drunk. At the time of his marriage to a Scottish girl he worked at a local brickworks. His first son, William, was born in December, 1904, and his second son, John, was born in August, 1907. While Higgins drank his way through his wages of 24 shillings a week his family suffered terrible hardship. His wife had to work, and in 1910, weak and undernourished, she died. Higgins claimed Poor Law relief, but instead of using it to maintain his two boys he spent it on drink.

The workhouse authorities, made aware of what was happening to the two children, told Higgins he would have to pay for their support or go to jail. The widower chose jail, and was discharged on August 24th, 1911. Two days later he picked up the boys from the Dysart workhouse and took them to Broxburn, where he persuaded a friend, Mrs. Elizabeth Hynes, to look after them. He continued to work at the brickyard, but lived the life of a tramp, sometimes sleeping in the woods, sometimes in a shed at the brickworks. He cooked his meals on an open fire, and was said to use his spade as a frying pan and his bucket as a soup plate.

Not surprisingly, the disreputable Higgins never

paid Mrs. Hynes a penny for his children's keep, and in chagrin she went along to the workhouse inspector to complain. The inspector went to the brickworks to meet Higgins.

"You have to pay for the bairns, every week till they're old enough to support themselves," he said. "If you don't I'll take them back to the workhouse and you'll go back to prison for a much longer stretch this time."

Higgins evidently took some alarm at this, and picking up the two boys from Mrs. Hynes's house he went off to the brickworks with them and settled them in his shed there. Next day, a bitterly cold November day, the brickworks foreman stopped at the shed and shook his head dolefully at the two little mites, crouched in the straw in a corner.

"You can't stay here with those wee bairns, Patrick," the foreman said. "They'll never last the winter in a place like this. You'll have to find them somewhere decent to live."

Higgins, intoxicated and shambling, did not reply. But his terrible plan must already have been forming in his drink-crazed mind. The boys stayed all day in the shed, and that evening their father somehow managed to give them a meal of Scotch broth – the last they would ever eat. As soon as they had finished the father and his two docile sons set out in the darkness across the moors. One man remembered them going, a miner named Hugh Shields.

Shields was in the village pub when later that night Higgins came in alone.

"What have you done with your wee bairns?" the miner asked at once.

"I've arranged for a friend to put them on the next ship to Canada," Higgins said. "I cannot afford to keep them – they'll be much happier in Canada."

Next day another miner, James Daly, noticed that

the two boys had gone from the brickworks shed. He asked Higgins what had happened to them.

"I met two ladies on a train," Higgins explained. "They had no children of their own, so they asked me if they could adopt them. I thought the bairns would be much happier with them, so I let them go."

Another miner, Alexander Fairnie, asked the same question. "They went off with a relative to another part of Scotland and were accidentally drowned," Higgins told him. And a shocked Mrs. Hynes, who met Higgins in the street, was told, "The wee laddies went off to Canada with a friend of mine and were drowned in a boating accident."

The police interviewed all these witnesses, an official at Dysart workhouse identified the boys' shirts, and the police even traced a woman who remembered giving the two boys their meal of Scotch broth. Higgins was arrested at a lodging-house in Broxburn at two o'clock in the morning. He made no protest as he was taken to jail; indeed, he had very little to say about the appalling murder of his children.

At his trial in Edinburgh Higgins claimed that anyone could have murdered the children – the case against him was based only on suspicion. To this he added a special defence that if he did kill the children he was mad, because he had a medical history of epilepsy. The judge's direction was that there was sufficient proof that Higgins was the murderer, so the verdict depended on whether or not the jury thought he was of unsound mind at the time. The jury decided he was not mad, and found him guilty, with a recommendation for mercy based on the lack of medical evidence about Higgins's state of mind at the time of the murder, which had happened two years previously. The recommendation was ignored. Before Higgins was hanged on Wednesday, October 1st,

1913, he told the prison chaplain that the sentence was just, and that drink had been his downfall.

10

BULLETS AND GUNS

The defendant said he liked to see how fast he could draw a gun. "It's a hobby with me. Some people take up golf. I took up guns."

Today we are almost used to criminals carrying guns, and even policemen returning fire. But midway through the twentieth century the thought of a single pistol being aimed in anger was enough to spark off newspaper stories of Chicago-style violence. When it occurred for the first time in Britain a Scotland Yard official said, "This is the start of a new era in crime. We've been worried about it. Now it has happened."

The new crime was armed robbery. The first time it made headlines was when Alec de Antiquis was shot dead in a London street in 1947.

Until then, the streets of London were safe. Passers-by could be relied upon to tackle fleeing raiders without fear of ending up as target practice. Scotland Yard even encouraged bystanders to "have a go" at bandits. But behind this official complacency a new breed of criminal was emerging – shiftless, brutal young thugs with a contempt for "old-fashioned coppers" and law-abiding citizens alike. They had grown up during the war, often without proper parental control, and had drifted into a get-rich-quick spivvery which was a feature of the otherwise austere life of the 1940s.

One of them was 23-year-old Charles Henry

Jenkins, a small-time gang leader. Armed with pistols, his mobsters raided a jeweller's shop in the Bayswater Road and got away with loot worth £5,000. But one of the gang, Bill Walsh, double-crossed the others and ran off with the takings.

Jenkins, broke, decided to try another stick-up. With two of his associates, Christopher Geraghty, 20, and Terence Rolt, 17, he attacked a jeweller's shop in Charlotte Street, off Tottenham Court Road. A shot was fired into the wall, but the staff reacted so violently that the bandits were forced to flee empty-handed. Outside the shop de Antiquis, father of six children, summed up the situation and swung his motor-cycle into the path of the bandits, shouting and waving an arm. There was a shot, and he fell dying.

The legendary Spilsbury was called in for the post-mortem, but he was a shadow of his former self, a sick and unsure old man. Puzzled and confused, he probed the exit wound of the bullet, unaware that it had dropped from the dead man's head on to the floor. Tactfully, an assistant said, "You've found it, Sir Bernard." But the old man knew his powers had gone. It was his last case – eight months later he committed suicide.

A few days after the shooting an eight-year-old boy found a revolver on the Thames foreshore at Wapping. It was a .320 loaded with five large cartridges and a spent case. Three of the rounds had misfired. Ballistics expert Robert Churchill identified the gun as the one which had killed Alec de Antiquis. Then another gun – a .455 Bulldog revolver loaded with four live rounds and one empty case – was found nearby by another boy. Churchill decided this was the gun which had fired the shot into the wall of Jays' jewellery shop. Both guns were identified as having been stolen during a raid on a gunsmith's shop a couple of days before the Bayswater Road robbery.

A Southend fence led police to Bill Walsh, who in turn named Jenkins and Geraghty. After their arrest it didn't take too long to squeeze out the name of the third member of the Charlotte Street gang, Terence Rolt. Geraghty finally confessed to killing de Antiquis. His stolen revolver was fired for the last time at the Old Bailey, where all three men stood trial for murder. Asked to demonstrate how quickly he could fire the weapon, Robert Churchill pointed it dramatically at the ceiling and squeezed the trigger four times in rapid succession. The clicks were heard right across the hushed courtroom.

Geraghty, Jenkins and Rolt were found guilty of murder. On Friday, September 19th, Geraghty and Jenkins were hanged at Pentonville Prison. Because of his youth, Rolt was sentenced to be detained during His Majesty's pleasure.

The science of ballistics, by which the bandits' two guns were identified, is the simplest and oldest of all the forensic sciences. It is especially used to link firearms with the bullets they fire. All gun barrels leave distinctive marks on their bullets, and once a firearm is found it can be said with absolute certainty whether or not a bullet fired into someone came from that particular gun – the bullet, so to speak, bears the "fingerprints" of its gun barrel. The distinctive marks on a bullet come particularly from the rifling grooves found inside gun barrels – they are designed to make the bullet spin on its axis so as to increase its speed and force.

When a forensic pathologist studies a firearm wound he must decide whether this is an accident, suicide, or murder.

By studying the inlet and exit holes, he can deduce the direction of fire, the angle, and the range. A bullet striking the surface at right angles makes a clean hole in the skin about its own diameter, or perhaps even smaller, because of the elasticity of the skin. The skin stretches in front of the bullet and when the bullet passes contracts to its normal state. The bullet-hole is left with a sort of rim, where the surface of the skin has been removed – this rim distinguishes an inlet from an exit hole. If the bullet strikes at an angle the hole is oval, but the rim is still there. The exit hole usually shows only tearing and puckering outwards of the edges, with perhaps small bits of bone which may have been driven along the line of fire.

In the case of a suicide, or murder at point-blank range, when a firearm is held with its muzzle against the skin the rush of compressed gases and their subsequent expansion tears the skin, often in a cross-shape, and the wound is much larger than the bullet. The tissues around and inside the wound are distinctively blackened. In the case of suicide the victim sometimes drops the weapon, and sometimes it is grasped in the victim's hand by cadaveric spasm. No murderer can place a weapon in the hand of his victim and cause it to be firmly grasped, although many a murderer has tried to simulate suicide in this way.

Bullets have enormous destructive power, but sometimes the effects of shooting are bizarre. In a case reported in 1951 a man suffering from depression came down to breakfast in his kitchen with blood trickling from a wound in each temple. He began to eat the meal as if nothing had happened. His wife called a doctor and it was deduced that the previous evening he had shot himself with a .38-inch revolver. He got up in the morning, washed, brushed his hair, dressed himself, and cooked his own breakfast, all the time perfectly conscious. He recovered completely, but remembered nothing of his attempted suicide.

In another case a man who had died suddenly in 1953 was examined at Guy's Hospital and cause of death was given as the rupture of an aneurysm of the aorta. A hole in the aorta led to a large sac filled with an old blood clot. Inside the clot was a lead ball of the type used in shrapnel of the First World War. The man had a scar on his left shoulder, and there was no exit wound. He was discharged from the army in 1916 as a result of shrapnel wounding. He got a job in an office where he worked for 35 years, always in the best of health. At the age of 55 he said he felt tired, collapsed and died from the effects of his wound.

Although ballistics (a term meaning the study of projectiles in flight, which is only part of the task of a firearms examiner) has been used to link guns to bullets for two centuries, the first case in which ballistics evidence was used in a court case in Britain occurred after the shooting of a policeman in 1927. The victim was discovered by a farm worker in Stapleford Abbots, Epping Forest, at dawn on Tuesday, September 27th. and identified as the village bobby, PC George Gutteridge. He had been shot twice in the chest and once in each eye.

There had been a number of burglaries recently in the village, and it seemed from the scene-of-crime evidence that Gutteridge had stopped a motorist and was questioning him when he was shot. The motorist, it was thought, had stolen the car, for a local doctor, Edward Lovell, almost immediately reported that his new Morris car was missing from his garage. Later the car was found abandoned in South London. There was blood that matched that of the dead policeman on the front seat and on the floor there was a Webley .455 revolver bullet-case, Mark IV pattern. The four bullets removed from the policeman's body were all .455 calibre, and all had distinct rifling marks.

Several months later another car was stolen in South London, near the place where Dr. Lovell's Morris was found abandoned. Police were tipped off that the car thief was one William Kennedy, who carried a gun.

Kennedy was traced to Liverpool where police had to lay siege to his home before they could arrest him. Hard though it is to believe today, Detective Inspector John Kirschner, of Scotland Yard, who interviewed Kennedy, was struck by the fact that Kennedy was a criminal who used a car and carried a gun, just as the killer of PC Gutteridge had used a car and carried a gun – the point being that motoring gunmen were then so rare that they stood out from the criminal crowd. Kennedy then implicated his accomplice, a South London garage-owner named Frederick Browne.

At Browne's garage police found four revolvers, one of them a Webley .455, and a stock of Mark IV pattern bullets. The two men were put on trial at the Old Bailey, where Robert Churchill's ballistic evidence roundly condemned them. He told the jury that he had test-fired Browne's .455 Webley and the rifling marks on the bullets were exactly identical to those on the bullets taken from PC Gutteridge's body. He and a group of army officers from Woolwich Arsenal had then test-fired more than a thousand .455 Webley revolvers to see if the rifling marks matched the bullets taken from PC Gutteridge – none of them were identical. He also showed that the breech face and firing pin of Browne's revolver had produced rifling marks identical to those found on the base of the cartridge found in Dr. Lovell's car. Mark IV pattern ammunition for .455 Webley revolvers had been declared obsolete by the British Army early in the First World War because it was packed with black powder – this had been replaced by a newer type of propellant. Traces of the black powder had been found in PC Gutteridge's eye wounds. Browne and Kennedy were found guilty and hanged on May 31st, 1928.

In the days before the government's clamp-down on

owning hand-guns daredevil Jack Day, a 30-year-old car salesman, once owned 177 swords and firearms. He was a fanatical collector, and as is the case with many another fanatical collector, guns were his undoing.

Day lived with his wife Margaret in Edward Street, Dunstable. The Days frequently employed a local girl, Patricia Dowling, as their baby-sitter, and on Tuesday, August 23rd, 1960, Patricia was joined on duty by her friend Mary Davies. Soon after eight o'clock that evening Mrs. Margaret Day arrived home alone. Instead of paying off Patricia there and then, she asked the baby-sitter if she would mind slipping around the corner to buy a frozen pork pie. Patricia willingly agreed, and on the way to the shop Mary Davies – who had gone with her – dropped off at her own home.

Patricia bought the pie and returned to the Days' house in Edward Street. The trip to the pie shop and back had taken her about ten minutes, she thought. She had no need to knock, because she had left the front door ajar. When she went in through the living-room she saw at once that Margaret Day had a visitor. This man, she subsequently learned, was Keith Arthur. She remembered that the man looked at her and made a remark about a pendant she was wearing, and then they talked about a bracelet on his wrist. Arthur said something to the effect that every link in his bracelet was nine-carat gold, and Patricia and Mrs. Day didn't believe him. While they were still talking about the bracelet Patricia looked through a rear window and saw Jack Day coming into the house through the back. At that moment Mrs. Day was sitting down and Keith Arthur was standing near her.

According to Patricia, when Jack Day came into the room he said to Keith Arthur, "What are you doing here?"

"The way he said it, I thought they were going to

fight or something. Then Mr. Arthur said, 'I came to see if you would buy me a drink, Jack,' or something like that. Mr. Day then said, 'This will go with it,' or something similar, and pulled a gun from his pocket. I heard a bang and saw a flash and then I ran home."

Day was already known to police, not through any criminal activity but because of his daredevil nature. He had been a dirt-track rider, and had a reputation as a heavy drinker and a fast driver. He had once been reported to the police as owning a .38 Enfield revolver, for which he was not registered, but the police were unable to find the weapon. He had recently disposed of his formidable arsenal of weapons, but his appetite for shooting remained as keen as ever.

The lethal ingredient added to this dangerous cocktail was that he was not very bright. It was later to be said on his behalf that he had the mind of a child, and was "lacking in normal balance, sense of proportion and responsibility."

He had apparently gone on record as having said he would shoot anyone who had an affair with his wife. His friend Keith Arthur wasn't present when that was said, and had he been it might have served as a warning, for Arthur often boasted about his affairs with women.

On August 25th, 1960, the day after the confrontation between the two friends in Day's living-room, Farmer Tony Sinfield and his wife Enid were baling hay in one of their fields on Dunstable downs when, pausing to lean on his pitchfork, Mr. Sinfield noticed a man's jacket lying in a bed of nettles near an outhouse.

"Never seen that before," he grunted, and together he and his wife went over to the jacket. It was then that they noticed a shoe protruding from behind some sacks. The farmer bent to pick up the shoe – and discovered it contained a human foot. Gingerly he pulled away the sacks, and there before him lay the body of a man, lying on his back.

The man's identity was established as soon as the police were on the scene. In his inside pocket they found an army pay-book in the name of Keith Arthur.

Arthur was a machine operator who worked in a local factory. He also bought and sold second-hand cars. He was married with two children, and like his friend Jack Day had a reputation in Dunstable as something of a heavy drinker. He died, said Dr. Francis Camps, the pathologist who carried out the post-mortem, from a single gunshot wound, but had been killed elsewhere and taken to the vicinity of the outhouse on Mr. Sinfield's farm.

Detective Superintendent Dennis Hawkins, called in from Scotland Yard to lead the murder hunt, decided that because the body had been well concealed, and the outhouse was hidden from the road by thick hedgerows, the killer must be a local man, and that "elsewhere" must be somewhere in Dunstable. Dozens of police officers scoured the fields for the murder weapon, but they failed to find it. Convinced that the man he was after was somewhere in the town, Hawkins put every officer in Dunstable on the alert.

Convinced too that sooner or later one of them would find the killer, Hawkins waited. The lead he wanted came when a policewoman met Patricia Dowling's mother and heard the story of the shooting incident at Jack Day's house. The day after Keith Arthur's body was found, Day was arrested in a police swoop on the Horse and Jockey pub in Dunstable. While he was held in custody a mountain of evidence was built up against him. Blood on his clothes was found to be the same group as Keith Arthur's, and soil and debris on his trousers matched samples taken at the farm outhouse where the body was found. And in the storeroom at the garage where he worked the police found the .38 Enfield with which he killed Arthur.

It looked like a cut and dried case of murder. But the first indication that it might not be like that at all came when Day decided to make a written statement. He said:

"I came home from the Horse and Jockey, parked my car and went indoors. Keith was there. I hadn't seen him for some time. I said 'Hello' to him, like you know. I went to take my clothes off as I got indoors. The wife and the baby-sitter were there. That is why I cannot understand how it happened. I took my gun out of my pocket. It was in a handkerchief. I put the gun down on the settee. The next thing I knew the damned thing went off! Keith was sort of standing there. I said, 'Blimey, sorry it happened.' He said, 'It has got me in the throat.' He looked as if he had been scratched like, everything happened quick. I gave him my handkerchief to put on it. I had two handkerchiefs, one on the gun, and another in my pocket."

Incredibly, Day then claimed that he and Arthur, who was losing blood heavily and could hardly walk, went into Dunstable town centre looking for someone to help.

"We went to see if we could find a doctor down the town. We got as far as the milk bar and Keith collapsed. No one came to give us a hand, but he was choking, you know, and coughing out blood out of his mouth. I got my arm around him and we rushed home. I ran all the way down to the Square to get my car, that's the Square near the public conveniences. When I got back Keith was laying in a pool of blood in the kitchen. I picked him up and took him through to put him in the car. He was dead when I got him in the car. I just panicked and I didn't know what to do. I don't know how I got him in the car. I didn't know what to do with him so I dropped him in that old shed up the top there. I just grabbed any old thing to cover him. I knew they would find him. It was dark. I expected to find you [the police] when I got back. The wife told me to give myself up but I daren't. That is the truth.

"I wrapped the gun up the following day and the ammunition I got with it. You can go and pick it up now. I knew you must find out anyway. It's in the spares building at Stansbridge Motors."

The "old shed" referred to in the statement was Farmer Sinfield's outhouse, where Day dumped his friend's body. He was familiar with the place because he was a relative of the Sinfields.

Jack Day was brought to trial at Bedfordshire Assizes in January, 1961, where gun experts testified that the distance between the revolver and the injury to Keith Arthur's throat was a maximum of nine inches. As we have seen, when a revolver is fired within an inch or two of the skin, the hot gases which emerge with the bullet enter the tissues and expand, causing the skin to tear. Most of the powder is found inside the tissues, but there are often traces of blackening, burning and "tattooing" around the entrance point. If the gun is fired at more than a couple of inches from the skin the effect of the hot gases vanishes and the entrance wound looks like a hole which might be caused by pressing a pencil-point into the tissues. The hole is round, with the characteristic rim already referred to, and surrounded by an area of singeing, blackening, and "tattooing." If all these signs are close together around the entrance hole, the indication is that the gun has been fired within a few inches of the skin. Beyond that range the marks diminish quickly. After a range of two feet nothing but the grease ring is likely to be seen.

This expert knowledge of what happens in a close-range shooting was going to be of vital importance to the prosecution. Jack Day's life hung on those few inches governing where the gun was actually held in relation to Keith Arthur's throat.

A defence ballistics expert agreed with the prosecution expert that the gun required great strength to fire it – as much as a pressure of 5 lbs on the trigger. The experts agreed too that it was impossible for the gun to go off by accident. One of them, Randolph Murray, added, "The Enfield .38 is the safest revolver in the world."

Giving evidence, Day told the court that on the day of the killing he had a day off. He stopped off for a drink at lunch-time, then went to the pictures and afterwards to the Horse and Jockey. All the time his revolver, fully loaded, was in his pocket. He habitually carried it around with him because his wife did not like guns left in the house. Most of the time it was carried in the door pocket of his car.

In the Horse and Jockey he met some people who knew he had guns. They talked about tricks with guns and about Russian roulette. One person there didn't believe that Day could play Russian roulette, and he bet him £1 that he couldn't.

"I demonstrated how to do it and how safe it is to do it," Day said. What he showed his saloon bar audience was that if one bullet is put in the chamber of a revolver which is working normally, and the chamber is then spun, the weight of the single bullet will ensure it will rest at the bottom of the chamber, so that theoretically pulling the trigger after the spin has stopped is perfectly safe.

Day then showed how he wrapped his handkerchief around the gun to store it tightly in his pocket. After he had a few drinks he came out of the pub and saw the police waiting outside.

"I knew they were trying to catch me on a drunken-driving charge," he said. "It annoyed me." He drove home, still feeling very annoyed about the police. He was thinking about going to the police station to complain about them because, he said, in the last two months they had been outside the public house every time he came out after a drink. He had reported this once before, but the police said they knew nothing about it.

The judge asked him if he realised that if the police had followed him they would have found a loaded revolver on him, and he replied, "Yes, sir, but I didn't think about that."

When he arrived home that evening he went through the back of the house into the living-room and saw Pat the baby-sitter standing in front of the door. He did not quite recall what he said to Keith Arthur when he first saw him in the room, but he thought it was something like, "How are you?" Asked by Mr. C. W. Abrahams, junior prosecution counsel, if he had said, "What are you doing here?" to Arthur, he replied, "It may be perfectly true, sir, I may have said that."

He remembered Arthur saying, "I have come to see if you'll buy me a drink, Jack." Day maintained that he then replied, "It depends on what you want to go with it." This reply, he said, was a standing joke between them, indicating whether Day could afford to buy him a chaser, and Arthur would know by that remark how he was "fixed" at the time. It was Day's custom when he drank a glass of beer to follow it with a glass of spirits whenever he could.

Day said he then began to unbutton his coat. "I pulled the handkerchief with the gun in it from my pocket. As I pulled the handkerchief off the gun it went off. I don't know how or why. I wasn't looking at Keith when the gun went off. To my knowledge I didn't touch the trigger."

He remembered that after the shot Pat was standing

near the door with her hands over her ears. His wife was sitting in a chair – as the gun went off "her mouth dropped open." Out of the corner of his eye he saw Arthur spin round. "I thought I said 'Sorry,' or something like that," Day said. "Arthur shook his right hand and put his other hand to his shirt. He said, 'It's got me through the shirt,'" then walked across the room and sat down. He took his hand away and there seemed hardly a mark there – it seemed like a graze. I said to him, 'It's just grazed you.'"

Arthur went to get a handkerchief out of his pocket but before he could find it blood was coming through his fingers. Day said, "We'd better go to the doctor's." They went out together and began to walk to Dr. Pinkerton's surgery. Because it was dark he couldn't see how badly Arthur was injured until they reached a zebra crossing in the High Street. Then Arthur collapsed on the ground beside him.

"He was in a terrible state," Day said. "There was blood all over the pavement. I was really worried by this time. I picked him up and said, 'Come on, Keith, we'll go down to the hospital.'" He told Arthur to wait there while he ran back to fetch his car. By this time Arthur was choking on his own blood.

Day put his arm around his friend's shoulder and helped him back home along Regent Street, half carrying, half dragging him. Arthur could hardly walk by this time, and he fell down a couple of times. He got the wounded man into his car and set off for the hospital. Arthur suddenly fell forwards on to the floor of the car.

"I saw his face then. I realised he was dead," Day said. "I think it was then that I went to pieces. It's a job to explain what I did next. I wanted to get rid of him, but I didn't want to. I think that's why I went up to the farm outhouse, because I thought someone would find him up there. I don't remember much about the ride, but I remember opening the door and picking him up. He fell from my hands on to the ground. I think I fell over him trying to pick him up."

He managed to drag Arthur to the outhouse. It was pitch-black there, but he knew the layout of the place because he used to go there when he was shooting.

"I seemed to go mad," he said. "I just dragged everything all over the place." He drove home after dumping the body, and his wife said to him, "How's Keith?" He replied. "He's dead."

His wife gave him the bullet. There was, he noted, very little damage on it. It was almost in perfect condition, and that didn't make sense to him. He put the cartridge case and the bullet together and put it in his pocket.

What didn't make sense to Day made a good deal of sense to the ballistics experts. High-velocity bullets fired at close ranges can fragment without striking any highly resistant body, probably from the effect of their own centrifugal force, but in many other cases the bullet passes through the body and exits the other side. How much damage is caused to it depends largely upon whether or not it strikes bone. In the case of Keith Arthur the bullet went through his throat, a narrow part of the body, and, missing any bone, exited cleanly. All the medical evidence suggests that after that he bled to death.

Why didn't Day take his injured friend to the ambulance station, he was asked. He replied, "I knew there was no one there. At least I have never seen anyone there. It is always dark at night." He thought he could get Arthur to hospital quicker in his own car.

Cross-examined, he said he used to practise shooting in a field with a revolver strapped to his side. He liked to see how fast he could draw a gun. "It's a hobby with me," he said. "Some people take up golf. I took up guns." He described how he would shoot pigeons sitting on walls through his car window, and said he had once killed a fox with a .45 revolver. The judge asked him, "Are you telling the jury that in case you saw a pigeon on a wall you carried a revolver to shoot out of the car window?"

When Day replied, "Yes," the judge said, "What about the people on the other side of the wall?"

Day replied, "I mean in the country."

He was not jealous of his wife, he said. Asked about the remark that he would shoot anyone he caught with his wife, he said, "I don't remember having made such a remark. It isn't the type of remark I make."

During his evidence Day complained bitterly about his arrest at the public house. The police "came in like a fire engine." One gripped his right am, another his left arm, and another ran his hands all over him. "They came through the door in a rush. One pulled a wallet out of my pocket. Everyone was standing there and staring. The only thing that gets my back up is when I have any dealings with the police. I once told them that any time that they thought I was intoxicated I would take them from A to B in perfect safety in a car."

Dr. Rowland Hill said that in his view Day had always been incapable of following a life of steady, methodical and progressive routine, with a normal sense of serious purpose. "I found him lacking in normal balance, sense of proportion and responsibility," he said.

So was it all a terrible accident, as Day claimed, or was it deliberate? The only other witness to the incident was Day's wife Margaret. Aware that her evidence was to be vital, a hushed courtroom watched her go, hatless and wearing a fur coat, into the witness box and take the oath. She had, she said, no feelings for Keith Arthur. She didn't like him, and thought nothing of him. Even so, she thought he was a person who might like her. Before the night of the shooting he had never been to her house before without her husband being there at the same time. Asked if her husband was jealous of her, she said he was possessive. She had never tried to make him jealous or maintain his interest by pretending she had been out with other people.

On the night of the shooting, she said, her husband spoke first to Keith. "He said, 'What are you doing here?' – although I don't think they were his exact words. It wasn't in an angry voice, and I didn't sense there was trouble in his tone. Keith said he had come to see if Jack would buy him a drink. Jack made some remarks back to him. I believe he said, 'You have come after my wife.' It did sound then as if there might be trouble." At this point Mrs. Day broke down and sobbed, but quickly recovered.

When the gun went off, she said, Keith Arthur went to his knees. "Jack said to Keith, 'Get up and don't be silly.' Keith was supported by my husband out of the house. My husband was dragging Keith by the feet. I was in the house when they came back. They were gone about seven or eight minutes. They came to the back door. My husband said he was going to get his car to take Keith to the hospital. At this time Keith was on the kitchen floor. I looked around the living-room and found a bullet under the table. One of the walls was grazed, so I put an extra piece of wallpaper of the same pattern over the mark.

"My husband came back at about ten-fifteen. I asked him where Keith was. At that time I didn't know he was dead. My husband replied, 'I have just dug his grave.' I told him to go to the police. After that we had no further conversation about it."

She was asked about an earlier witness who had said that Mrs. Day had told her she used to make her husband jealous by dressing up so that it looked as if she had been out. Mrs. Day replied she had never said anything like that. Nor did she remember her husband threatening anyone he found with her, "but he might have done." When the gun went off she did not see a handkerchief, nor did she find one in the room afterwards. At the sound of the explosion she panicked and ran out into the hall.

Patricia Dowling, the 13-year-old baby-sitter, said that when Day spoke to Arthur, she thought he didn't sound very happy, and she thought there was going to be a fight.

Mr. John Hobson QC, MP, summing-up for the prosecution, said it was the Crown's case that Day shot Arthur in a temper. There were two things that made Day's explanation quite unacceptable. The first thing was that the revolver could scarcely have gone off by accident. Even though a handkerchief might possibly pull back the cocking piece, it would still not mean that the gun would fire unless a pressure of 5 lbs was placed on the trigger. There was also the evidence of two experts that the wound in Arthur's throat was caused by a weapon that was discharged at a maximum distance of nine inches. At no stage in his story had Day said anything which would bring the revolver this close.

"When Arthur collapsed in the street, why didn't Day take him to the ambulance station?" he asked. "Perhaps a test of Day's veracity may be made about the point whether he pulled Arthur from the house with his arms under Arthur's armpits. Mrs. Day said that he was dragged out by the feet."

Mr. Arthur James QC, defending, said there were two accounts of what happened – what the girl Pat had said and what the accused had said in his statement. He thought that at one stage the prosecution were setting out to show that Pat had seen the gun withdrawn from the pocket of Mr. Day without any handkerchief covering it. But the evidence fell far short of that. The girl had only said, "I can't remember back over five months. I wasn't particularly interested in what people were doing or what they were saying, but I heard certain words spoken." She had told the court, "I heard Mr. Day say, 'What are you doing here?' in a tone which she thought was angry, and she edged towards the door.

Mr. James commented, "That is the evidence of the prosecution, but are you to determine this matter on the evidence and recollection of one young girl as to her interpretation of the tone of this man's voice?"

Jack Day maintained an air of supreme disinterest in his trial. Frequently he broke into bouts of laughter, causing the judge to remind him of the seriousness of the matter. It took the all-male jury just 20 minutes to find him guilty of murder. Asked if he had anything to say before being sentenced, he replied, "No, only that I am not guilty, sir. I didn't pull the trigger."

Day's mother was dragged screaming from the court as she shouted at the judge, "You have sentenced an innocent man. You will regret it." Then she fainted.

The gallows at Bedford Prison were about 50 yards from the death cell, and as he was being led to them by hangman Harry Allen and his assistant Henry Robson, Day turned to them and said, "I'm sorry I did it. I didn't really want to kill him."

Daredevil Jack Day had often boasted that he would not live beyond 30. That was his exact age when he was hanged.

11

POISON, THE SILENT KILLER

The managing director was delighted with his new recruit. He had no way of telling that the eager young fellow was stark raving mad

Murder by poisoning is murder by stealth – there is no mess of blood and bone, no firearm wounds, no hands gripping necks or pulling on ligatures. Poisoners generally do not hide bodies or dismember them, rather, they stand back from their evil work and let the forensic pathologist decide whether it is murder, accident or suicide, for plenty of people kill themselves deliberately or accidentally by taking poison. Because it is not "hands-on" killing, poisoning has been favoured by many middle-class murderers. An analysis of murder in Britain over the last century might well prove that artisans and working-class people did most of the stabbing and strangling, while white-collar workers and women – like Seddon, Armstrong, Crippen and Adelaide Bartlett — did most of the poisoning.

There are scores of poisons which can end human life, but several particularly have been favoured by murderers – they include strychnine, antimony, arsenic. phosphorus, and prussic acid. All of them bring about an agonising death. Another poison, thallium, was the chosen method of Britain's most notorious poisoner, Graham Young, who killed for his own perverted pleasure. Thallium had never been used in a British murder case before Graham Young, which is why it took such a long time to identify the illnesses of his victims.

Symptoms of thallium poisoning are hair-loss, waves of severe abdominal pains, diarrhoea, vomiting, haemorrhage, and great sensitivity to touch – a victim cannot, for instance, bear the touch of bedsheets on his flesh. Convulsions and coma precede death.

Thallium is a soft, white metallic element used mostly today in making paint, glass, dyes and optical lenses. But in the past it has had a volatile and dangerous career as a medicine. Towards the end of the nineteenth century small doses were recommended as a treatment for ringworm, but the side-effects were evidently so startling that its use was abandoned. Unfortunately, it was revived for its therapeutic properties in the 1920s, and became widely used in treating ringworm in children. The side-effects of these minuscule doses – rashes, headache, muscular pains in the legs – were generally understood but thought to be worth the end result.

That, however, was not the view which prevailed in Granada in 1930, when 16 schoolchildren suffering from ringworm were treated with thallium acetate. Almost immediately they developed headaches, breathing problems, acute stomach pains, dimness of vision and a host of other ill-effects. Only two of them were to survive. The first death occurred after only two days; there were four more deaths on the fifth day, three on the sixth, and the other five died in the next ten days.

Used in a proprietary brand of rat poison, thallium was employed by a Mrs. Fletcher in New South Wales in 1953 to murder her husband. After she had administered several doses his hair fell out, he had pains in the hands and feet, and he was nervous and crying. His condition was not diagnosed, and he died after 11 days. At the post-mortem half a grain of thallium was found in his body. Police began to suspect foul play when it was remembered that four years earlier Mrs. Fletcher's first husband died of similar undiagnosed symptoms. His body was exhumed, and substantial quantities of thallium were found in it. The case illustrates a vital point in favour of the killer – that by the time correct diagnosis is made (if indeed it is ever made) the poison has performed its deadly work. Then only a post-mortem can positively reveal what happened.

Armed with this knowledge, 23-year-old Graham Young went to work at John Hadfield's, manufacturers of photographic equipment, after undergoing a course at a Government Training Centre in 1971. The company's managing director, Godfrey Foster, was delighted with his new recruit – he reckoned Young was just the right sort of chap to fit in well as a junior storeman. He had no way of telling that the eager young fellow was stark raving mad.

For the new junior storeman had packed some fantastic experiences into his 23 years – including nine of them spent in Broadmoor. Graham Young was only 13 when he killed his stepmother with poison. Then he administered belladonna to his sister and antimony to his father and a school friend. Fortunately, Young wasn't yet as perfect a poisoner as he was to become, and all three recovered.

He was 14 when he stood in the dock at the Old Bailey. A doctor told the judge that the schoolboy was suffering from a psychopathic disorder, and it was extremely likely that he would kill again. The judge recommended that he should not be released for 15 years without the Home Secretary's permission. In fact he was released nine years later, in 1971.

One of the conditions was that he should live in a hostel in Slough, Buckinghamshire. While he was there he befriended Terry Sparkes, of Welwyn Garden City, who twice went back to Young's room for a glass of wine. After one such evening Sparkes felt a violent pain in the lower abdomen. He began to get seriously worried when his leg muscles seized up during a football match. He didn't play for the rest of that season, or the next. Subsequent events proved he was lucky to live to tell the tale, for Young was using him as a guinea pig for his experiments with poisons, dropped surreptitiously into those nocturnal glasses of wine.

The manager of the Government Training Centre at Slough knew Young had some sort of criminal record, but he didn't think it was necessary to advise Hadland's, the young man's new employers, about that. He couldn't have done so, anyway, because no one had told him any of the details. So on April 23rd, 1971, Graham Young started work for the first time in his life. During the next twelve months he was going to bring slow, agonising death to two of Hadland's employees and dreadful pain to four other equally innocent members of staff.

The day after he got his job at Hadland's, Young went to a Wigmore Street, London, chemist and bought 25 grams of antimony, signing "M.E. Evans" in the poisons register. "It's for qualitative and quantitative analysis," he explained to the chemist. Later, from the same chemist, and using the same name, he bought a quantity of thallium.

At Hadland's next day storeman Bob Egle called out, "Make some tea, will you, Graham?"

Young jumped to the task. With his back to his workmates he slipped some of his lethal powder into Bob Egle's tea. Slowly the storeman became ill. Three months after Graham Young started work, Bob Egle was admitted to hospital. That night Young told his cousin, with whom he was lodging, that his workmate was ill.

"He's got an obscure virus," Young said. "He's suffering from all sorts of aches and pains, and his hair's fallen out." Then he added prophetically, "He will lose the use of his legs eventually." Later he was to tell his cousin that he had been promoted to Mr. Egle's job.

A week after being admitted to hospital Bob Egle died. The doctors were bewildered. A post-mortem revealed nothing.

At Hadfield's the funeral arrangements were discussed under a pall of gloom. Managing director Godfrey Foster chose Young to attend with him, to represent the factory workers. "You were his closest associate," explained Mr. Foster.

On the way to the funeral with his boss, Young discussed his co-worker's illness in remarkably explicit medical terms, and although he hadn't seen the death certificate, diagnosed the cause of death that had been entered on it.

Young had killed Bob Egle with thallium, so he knew all the symptoms. He knew too that Bob Egle would not have noticed any different taste in his cup of tea – the highly poisonous salts of thallium are soluble, colourless, and nearly tasteless, and therefore easily administered. They can also operate through the skin by absorption. The poison is highly resistant – when Bob Egle was cremated his ashes were analysed, and thallium was found among them.

At the annual stock-taking at Hadlands, Graham Young eagerly volunteered to take care of refreshments and was given the keys of the tea room. He offered a cup of coffee to the managing director, who hesitated, then declined. Instead Young gave the coffee, laced with antimony, to a fellow-worker, Jethro Batt. After drinking only a mouthful and complaining of its bitter taste, Mr. Batt had violent pains, followed by sickness, loss of hair and hallucinations. "At one stage I contemplated suicide," he said afterwards.

Used for homicidal purposes, antimony comes in the form of a tartar emetic, a white powder which tastes metallic. A fatal dose causes difficulty in swallowing, a burning sensation in the throat, stomach pains, vomiting, and the hands, feet and face become bluish. There are accompanying cramps in the legs and calves, spasms, giddiness and black-outs. The victim becomes unconscious, and heart failure follows. The forensic pathologist will discover at post-mortem some of the same signs as in arsenic poisoning. In addition to that there will be considerable inflammation of the victim's lungs.

Young gave another cup of coffee, also laced with antimony, to Diane Smart, who soon developed the same symptoms as Mr. Batt. Then he decided to switch back to thallium. He chose as his victims Fred Biggs, aged 56, and his wife Anne, both Hadland's employees. One afternoon both were given drinks by Young while they worked in the storeroom.

That evening Fred Biggs left work feeling decidedly unwell. Next day he returned to work, and an apparently sympathetic Young asked him how he was feeling. When Mr. Biggs said the pains had gone Young handed him a cup of tea laced with thallium. Within hours Mr. Biggs was in severe pain. He was taken to hospital, and a tracheotomy was performed. His skin was scaling, and his hair could be plucked out easily. A few days later he died in the National Hospital for Nervous Diseases in London. The cause of death was given as poisoning.

While Fred Biggs was fighting for his life Graham Young wrote in his diary: "I have administered a fatal dose of the special compound and anticipate reports of his illness on Monday. He should die within a week. I gave him three separate doses; the total absorbed should be about 15 to 16 grams." A couple of days later he wrote: "He is surviving too long for my piece (sic) of mind." Another entry read: "It is better that he should die. It will be a merciful release for him, as if he should survive he will be permanently impaired."

Young's next victim, David Tilson, didn't drink too much of the cup of tea Young handed him because he thought it had been "wrongly sugared." But next day, a Saturday, he experienced a "pins and needles" feeling in his feet. The pain crept up his legs. After a weekend of acute discomfort he went to his doctor. Then his hair began to fall out. A bearded man with a lot of hair, he was taken to hospital, where a consultant said, "He looked like a three-quarters plucked chicken. He had hair-loss all over the place – beard, head, everywhere. It was very unusual. This made us think at once of heavy metals, and then of the possibility of thallium."

At this point Graham Young was beginning to get worried. He wrote in his diary, "I must consider this situation very carefully. If it looks like I'm going to be detected, then I shall have to destroy myself." He prepared an excess-of-fatal dose of thallium as his "exit" dose. But although he was to have ample opportunity to use it, he never did so.

At Hadfield's there was universal depression. Godfrey Foster, the managing director called in a team of medical experts, and at a staff meeting the workers were asked if they had any ideas about the illness in the factory. Young, puffing out his chest, asked the meeting's chairman, Dr. Arthur Anderson, "What about thallium? It's a very toxic metal. Thallious salts can be easily absorbed from mucous membranes of the mouth and gastro-intestinal tract, as well as from the skin."

Dr. Anderson was mildly surprised. Here was a very knowledgeable young storeman. The managing director quickly reassured him that thallium was not used at Hadfield's. It was then that the doctor gave it as his opinion that one option might be that someone was trying to poison the whole staff. Mr. Foster picked up a phone and called the police.

A routine police check on the past of the Hadland's staff didn't take long, and it soon brought Graham Young, the ex-Broadmoor poisoner, out of the woodwork. When he was arrested they even found thallium in his pocket. He told the police, "I suppose I had ceased to see them as people, or at least part of me had. They had become guinea pigs."

To one police officer he gave his theory on the illness of Jethro Batt, who was still in hospital. "His condition is believed to be caused by a form of heavy metal poisoning. If so, I would expect the hospital to use dynacatrol and potassium chloride." He refused to say what kind of poison he had given to Mr. Batt, although dynacatrol is an antidote for thallium poisoning.

Put on trial at St. Albans Crown Court, Young denied his confession. He said that while he was at Hadland's he had prepared a special compound containing thallium for "a fellow workmate and friend, Mr. Biggs" for use in his garden to get rid of insects. He was jailed for life – and life it really was. After serving 18 years he died in prison in 1990.

Poisoning by phosphorus, a non-metallic element, is comparatively rare. In the first half of the twentieth century the average number of deaths per year from phosphorus in Britain was six, most of which were suicides. The poison was used in rat-killer, and in wartime products like incendiary bombs and flares. It is not an easy poison for a murderer to use, because it has strong smell and unpleasant taste, as well as luminosity. Several post-war cases are on record of intended murderers having used it but failed to kill, and one, the case of Louisa Merrifield, where it was used and the victim died.

Louisa Merrifield, a rough-edged, hard-boozing Wigan lass of 46, had got herself a job as domestic servant to Sarah Ricketts, a widow of 79, who lived in a bungalow called Homestead on Blackpool's North Shore. Mrs. Merrifield lived in, sharing a bedroom at Homestead with her third husband Alfred. Mrs. Ricketts was evidently pleased with this arrangement, and began to talk about rewriting her will in favour of the Merrifields, rather than her first choice, the Salvation Army. What was in Mrs. Merrifield's mind after that might be gauged from the fact that she told three of her friends that an old lady had died and left her a bungalow worth £3,000. To one of them she said, "It was all left to me until that old bugger [her description of husband Alfred] got talking to her, and then it was left to us jointly."

In fact, while Mrs. Merrifield was doing all this talking Mrs. Ricketts was still very much alive. To another friend to whom she told the same story she confided, "Actually she's not dead yet, but she soon will be!"

One evening Mrs. Merrifield phoned Dr. Albert Wood, the local doctor, and asked him to come and see Mrs. Ricketts as she was ill.

"Can't it wait until the morning?" the doctor asked.

"Well, what happens if she dies in the night?" said Mrs. Merrifield.

The doctor decided to call, and found nothing wrong with the patient more than mild bronchitis. When he remonstrated with Mrs. Merrifield for calling him unnecessarily she replied, "I was frightened in case something happened to her during the night."

Next morning Mrs. Merrifield phoned the surgery again to say that Mrs. Ricketts was seriously ill. This time Dr. Woods was unavailable; his partner finally arrived at midday. He was both shocked and surprised at what he saw. The patient was dying, and there was nothing he could to save her. He called another doctor, but before he arrived Mrs. Ricketts was dead. Only 33 days had passed since the Merrifields moved in, and only 13 since the will was changed in their favour.

The post-mortem was conducted by Home Office pathologist Dr. G. B. Manning, who found four ounces of a dark brown fluid in Mrs. Ricketts's stomach – a mixture of brandy and rat poison. Although the brandy masked the taste of the rat poison, its distinct, garlic-like odour could still be smelt. His conclusion was that Mrs. Ricketts had died of poisoning by phosphorus, the most toxic of all the non-metallic elements. In fact it has much more similarity to arsenic and antimony in its ultimate action than it has to the non-metallic poisons

There was no sign of a half-empty tin of rat poison, the most likely source, despite an intensive police search. When the Merrifields candidly revealed that they were the sole beneficiaries of Mrs. Ricketts's will, they were arrested and brought to trial at Manchester Assizes on Monday, July 20th, 1953. In his summing-up Mr. Justice Glyn-Jones told the jury, "Murder by poison is a secret crime, and such murder is rarely if ever committed in the presence of eye-witnesses who can give you direct evidence of the administration of poison. It must therefore be established by circumstantial evidence, but that is not necessarily inferior to direct evidence."

The jury found Louisa Merrifield guilty of murder, and she was hanged at Manchester's Strangeways Prison on Friday, September 18th, 1953. They failed to agree on the case against her husband Alfred. At the next county assizes, where he was arraigned, the prosecution decided not to continue with the charge against him, and he was discharged. He received one-sixth of Mrs. Ricketts's estate, the rest going to the old widow's two daughters. He also received £500 for the Chamber of Horrors Waxworks Museum in Blackpool, for agreeing to have his effigy in wax standing by an effigy of his wife in their horror show.

Strychnine, a product of the tree *Strychnos nux vomica*, was the poison chosen by Frenchman Jean Pierre Vaquier to kill his English lover. Strychnine is a violent poison – it is unusual for a victim to live for more than two hours after a fatal dose. The first signs of poisoning are a sense of uneasiness and restlessness, together with a feeling of suffocation and sometimes a sense of impending doom. The facial muscles contract in a way that makes the victim seem to be grinning – a grin called the *risus sardonicus*. The head and limbs begin to twitch, and then come sudden tetanic convulsions violently affecting nearly all the body muscles. Arms and legs are stretched out stiffly, hands are clenched, the head is convulsively jerked backwards and forwards, the whole body becomes rigid, often in a bow-like shape. There is no control over the violent body movements, causing the victim to jerk across the floor unless restrained. The face becomes livid, the eyes are prominent and staring, and the victim gasps for breath. The convulsions last at the most for two minutes, then subside, leaving the victim exhausted. They can be brought on again by trivial happenings, like a sudden noise or an attempt to move. The spasms become more severe and last longer each time, until finally the victim dies in a state of utter exhaustion. Since throughout this entire terminal experience the victim's mind is quite clear, and he is totally conscious, strychnine poisoning is a particularly terrible way to die.

Jean-Pierre Vaquier, a wireless operator, met Mrs.

Mabel Jones when she was on holiday alone in Biarritz. Although he didn't speak a word of English and she didn't speak a word of French, they swiftly became lovers. What must have been like an early version of *Shirley Valentine* ended when Mrs. Jones got a telegram from her husband Alfred, landlord of the Blue Anchor in Byfleet, Surrey, asking her to come home. Thoroughly reconciled to the idea that the first mad affair in her nineteen years of marriage was behind her, she complied.

She had been back home only a couple of days when she received another telegram, this time from Vaquier. He had just arrived in London, he said. Mabel Jones' heart missed a beat, and taking advantage of a business trip that her husband had to make, she was soon reliving her holiday romance in bed with Vaquier in the Hotel Russell. At the end of a day and night she went sighing back to the Blue Anchor, happily accepting for a second time that her fling was finally behind her.

Hardly was she ensconced behind the bar, however, when there came a knock at the door. On the doorstep was the ubiquitous Vaquier, minus his luggage. "Do you have a room where I could stay?" he inquired haltingly.

If Alfred Jones when he came home was surprised to see this Frenchman in one of his guest rooms, he didn't show it. He accepted the explanation that Vaquier had come to England to try to sell a new type of sausage-making machine, and never remarked that that was an unusual occupation for a wireless operator. He shared his meals in complete amity with Vaquier, and didn't seem to mind that the new guest not only didn't pay for his lodgings but actually borrowed money from him.

On March 1st, 1924, a fortnight after he had settled himself in at the hotel-pub, Vaquier went off alone to

London. He called at a chemist's shop near Holborn and produced a list of chemicals which he said he needed for experiments he was doing on wireless. On the list was 100 grammes of chloroform, twenty grammes of perchloride of mercury, and .12 of a gramme of strychnine.

The chemist hesitated. He didn't know this customer, whose command of English was almost non-existent, and what the request amounted to was enough poison to kill twelve people. But Vaquier was persuasive, and reluctantly the chemist produced the poisons register for his signature. Vaquier signed himself "M. Wanker" – although it should be said in his defence that this pseudonym did not then enjoy the meaning in the lexicon of English vernacular which it commands today.

Another month went by, during which Vaquier became less and less welcome at the Blue Anchor. But he had his uses. On most nights a very drunk Alfred Jones had to be helped to bed, and the Frenchman frequently did this service for him. One such night occurred on March 29th, and when next day Jones came down to the bar he made at once for his bottle of bromo salts. He poured out a teaspoonful from the small quantity the bottle contained, stirred it into half a glass of water, and stared miserably at the result.

"These damned things won't fizz this morning," he remarked. Then he drank the solution at one gulp, and at once exclaimed, "Oh, God, they're bitter!"

At that moment Mrs. Jones came into the bar parlour. She picked up the bottle and studied its contents. Afterwards she recalled, "I moistened a finger, dipped it in the salts, and put it to my lips. The taste was extremely bitter. I noticed that the crystals were long and transparent. Bromo salts look quite different."

All this happened in a flash, and Mrs. Jones cried

out, "Oh, Daddy, they've been tampered with. Quickly! Someone get some salt and water!"

After swallowing the salt and water Jones was sick, and he was again sick after drinking a cup of strong tea containing common soda. He said, "I'm all right, but I'm going numb and feeling cold." Then the first acute spasm, which caused his body to bend backwards like a bow, occurred. Two members of his staff and Vaquier carried him up to his bedroom. A doctor arrived and asked to see the bottle. Mrs. Jones saw it had been moved in its position in the drawer, but as she handed it over she did not notice it had been washed out. Upstairs in his bed Jones was in a torment. Later that afternoon he died in dreadful agony.

Next day Mabel Jones challenged Vaquier: "You killed my husband!" He replied, "Yes, Mabs, for you."

A post-mortem established that Jones had died from strychnine poisoning. Grains of the salts which had fallen from the bottle when Jones mixed his drink were strychnine, and the empty bottle, although it had been washed, held traces of the poison.

The police moved Vaquier to another hotel, and Fleet Street crime reporters arrived in a swarm to interview him. He posed for pictures, then thrust a sheaf of papers at one reporter. "This is my life story," he whispered. "Your newspaper shall like it. It shall be yours if they pay me what I want for it ..." Then, in an even lower voice, he outlined a plan of escape to France, in which the reporter would convey him to the Kent coast in a fast car while the police weren't looking. When the photograph of Vaquier duly appeared in the next day's paper one reader who immediately recognised it was the Holborn chemist who had so reluctantly sold strychnine to the Frenchman in March.

Vaquier was arrested and charged. He was so short

that when he appeared in the dock at Surrey Assizes at Guildford in July, 1924, only his head and shoulders came above the dock rail. He declared that he was in no way involved in the death of Alfred Jones. But he did more than just admit to buying the chemicals. For, he said, he bought .25 of a gramme of strychnine, much more than the quantity mentioned by the chemist. He also bought 100 grammes of chloroform.

"Why did you buy the strychnine?" Sir Henry Curtis-Bennett QC, prosecuting, asked him.

"I was asked to do so by the solicitor of Mrs. Jones," he replied. He could not recall the solicitor's name, but he remembered that the poison was wanted for putting down a dog with the mange. He was asked why the solicitor could not have bought the poison for himself, and he replied, "He told me he was very busy and didn't have time to buy it."

Sir Patrick Hastings QC, defending, asked him, "Did the solicitor tell you to sign a false name in the register?"

"Yes."

"What do you mean by this sentence in your statement: 'I will make known tomorrow who administered the poison'? Who is the person you intended to name?"

"The solicitor of Mrs. Jones, who asked me to buy the poison."

Mrs. Jones' solicitor was then called to the witness box, and indignantly denied that there was a single word of truth in Vaquier's evidence.

Vaquier screamed in French from the dock when the jury found him guilty: he was innocent, his trial had been unfair, he could not be hanged. He had to be carried to the cells. There was little doubt about his guilt, but his motive remains something of a mystery. His object was not mercenary, for it was never suggested that either he or Mrs. Jones would benefit by her husband's death. Vaquier was probably obsessed by a passion for the dead man's wife, and had some vague idea that with Jones removed she might return to his arms. Against this it was proved that after his appearance at the Blue Anchor he never went to bed with Mrs. Jones and she never held out the slightest hope that he would. Indeed she made it clear that she never wanted Vaquier to come to England.

The little Frenchman was executed at Wandsworth on Tuesday, August 12th, 1924. It was recorded that he died bravely.

Passion was also the reason why Charlotte Bryant murdered her husband, and the poison she chose was arsenic.

The commonest source of arsenical poisoning is the arsenious acid called white arsenic, which in one form is white and opaque, like flour, for which it has been mistaken with fatal results. Because it has little taste and no colour, it is easily mixed with food by anyone with murder in mind. Once it used to be combined with potash or soda to make fly-papers, and potential murderers then discovered that by soaking the fly-papers in water they could obtain a strong arsenical solution. This was the method of arsenic-extraction used by the notorious poisoner Frederick Seddon, hanged at Pentonville in 1912. Toxic effects have also resulted from the use of copper arsenite as a pigment in wallpapers and even fabrics.

In acute poisoning arsenic works on an empty stomach within ten minutes; on a full stomach the interval can be up to 12 hours. Usually, though, the period is from half an hour to an hour. A sensation of heat developing into a burning pain is felt in the throat and stomach, and this is quickly followed by uncontrollable vomiting. The victim suffers from intense thirst, but drinking is immediately followed by rejection of the swallowed fluid. The features become sunken, the skin moist and bluish, the pulse is feeble and the victim gasps for breath. There is persistent pain in the stomach and cramps in the calves and the legs. The victim may go into a coma before death, but consciousness is often maintained until the end.

The forensic pathologist recognises arsenical poisoning because the stomach is hugely inflamed and parts or the whole of its mucous membrane vary from dark red to bright vermilion. And as all crime students know, arsenic doesn't go away. After chronic poisoning the pathologist will find it in almost every part of the body, but mostly in the liver and the kidneys. Arsenic and antimony also tend to preserve the body tissues and attack the organisms of putrefaction.

Charlotte Bryant was exceedingly unattractive, illiterate, slightly retarded, and married to an impoverished farm labourer who, it was said, was not the father of all her five children. She was also frequently drunk. In her early thirties, she looked much older, yet for all that this unlikely sex object was much in demand among the menfolk of the little Dorset village of Coombe. Boredom, and the sheer necessity of earning some extra money to make ends meet, prompted her to turn to part-time prostitution, especially as she had always enjoyed sex for its own sake.

Unlike many prostitutes who are supposed to despise their customers, Charlotte's head was full of romantic dreams of meeting a man who would make her happy. The man she focused upon for this task was a gypsy vagrant named Leonard Parsons. He was living apart from his common-law wife and four children, in rooms in the village, when just before Christmas, 1933, Charlotte met him casually for the first time and immediately fell in love with him. Without consulting her husband, she invited him to have Christmas dinner with them.

Parsons was one of those men who is good company in any company, and by the end of the day Frederick Bryant not only wanted him to stay but invited him to move into the spare room. Within a few days the new lodger and Charlotte were lovers. It never seemed to occur to Frederick, though, that his wife was jumping into bed with Parsons from the moment he went off to work. Then one day he did find out. And although he had always condoned his wife's prostitution, he went berserk with rage.

He ordered the gypsy to leave at once, and Parsons slunk away. But three days later Charlotte received a telegram from her lover asking her to meet him. Because even so simple a message was beyond her powers of literacy, she showed it to her husband.

"I'll give him something to think about," rumbled Bryant. "You go along and meet him, and I'll come with you."

As the two former friends confronted each other at the rendezvous Bryant shouted, "You keep away from my wife, d'you hear? If you want to go tom-catting, you do it round some other woman." But Parsons wasn't so easily dissuaded. He began to reason, and the direction of the conversation changed. After a little while the two friends who had become enemies were friends again. They shook hands, and two days after that Parsons resumed his old status in the Bryant household and his regular place in Charlotte's bed. There she stroked his hair and told him how wonderful it would be if they could spend the rest of their lives together. At that Parsons's ardour began to cool. The idea of spending the rest of his life with Charlotte had never occurred to him, and now that it did he didn't think much of it.

Aware that he was slipping through her passionate grasp, Charlotte decided something must be done quickly. At that time weedkiller was kept in every farm labourer's garden shed, and it often contained arsenic – it was comparatively easy for country people to buy it. Charlotte went into Yeovil and bought a tin of arsenical weedkiller from a chemist's shop, signing the poison register with a cross. Clutching the green tin, she went home and laced her husband's lunch with its contents.

That afternoon Frederick Bryant was seized with violent stomach pains. Charlotte sent a child for the local GP, Dr. McCarthy, who was in no hurry to call. When he arrived in the evening he found the labourer complaining of cramp in his legs, and put it down to gastro-enteritis.

Bryant quickly recovered, returned to work, then went down with another bout of the same symptoms, all of which coincided with Parsons's sudden announcement that he was bored with living as a paying guest in the Bryants' cottage and was off to seek his luck elsewhere. Charlotte was now desperate. She had to get him back. The first thing was to make sure that her husband did not recover from the third attack of "gastro-enteritis."

That happened next day, and it was so severe that a worried Dr. McCarthy put Bryant on a special diet. A couple of days later, on Saturday, December 21st, 1935, Charlotte left her sick husband with a lunch she had prepared heavily supplemented with arsenic, and set out for Weston-super-Mare, where she had heard that her erstwhile lover was living in a gypsy camp. By the time she returned home, having failed to see Parsons, Bryant's condition had considerably worsened. Next day, Sunday, he was taken to the Yeatman Hospital, Sherborne, where he died within a few hours.

At the subsequent post-mortem conducted by Home Office pathologist Dr. Gerald Roche Lynch,

Bryant's body was found to contain more than four grains of arsenic. Police descended on Charlotte's cottage, bundling her and her children off to the workhouse while they searched the place inch by inch and dug up the entire garden. They found arsenical traces in the samples of dust and dirt carefully swept up in the cottage, but that wasn't enough to bring her to trial, since arsenic in one form or another was often kept in a farm labourer's cottage. They also found a battered, empty green-coloured tin of weedkiller in the garden, but there was no way of proving Charlotte had bought it.

Charlotte's eventual undoing was a woman friend, Mrs. Lucy Ostler, who told the police that once Mrs. Bryant had shown her a green tin, saying, "I must get rid of that." A few days later Mrs. Ostler had found the same tin in the ashes in the boiler, and had thrown it out into the backyard, where the police found it. Mrs. Ostler recounted how often Charlotte had told her she hated her husband, and how soon after Frederick's death Charlotte had suddenly said, "If they can't find anything they can't hang me." If there was a friend that Charlotte could have done without at that time it was Mrs. Ostler.

On the strength of this rather flimsy evidence Charlotte was arrested and put on trial at Dorchester Assizes, where the prosecution freely admitted that they had not been able to establish that she had bought arsenic in any form. But they had the evidence of Lucy Ostler, and also that of an insurance agent named Tuck, who testified that he had met Charlotte returning from the hospital after her husband's death. "He's gone," Charlotte told Tuck. "I've been a good wife to him – and no one can say I poisoned him."

Somewhat surprised, Tuck asked, "Why should they?"

"You never know what will come of these things,"

Charlotte replied cryptically.

Worse still for Charlotte was the evidence of Dr. Roche Lynch, who had analysed the ashes in the boiler.

"There were 149 parts of arsenic to the million," he said. "The expected concentration of arsenic in coal ashes in a domestic fire is about 45 parts per million. The large amount of arsenic in the Bryants' fire can only suggest that it was thrown into the fire by someone."

That decided it for the jury. Charlotte was found guilty and sentenced to death. But it wasn't quite over.

When her counsel, Mr. J. D. Caswell KC, arrived at his chambers the day after the sentencing he found a letter from Professor William Bone, of Imperial College, London. When the two men met later that day the professor told Mr. Caswell that Dr. Roche Lynch's evidence was inaccurate. It had been established that the proportion of arsenic normally found in the ashes of domestic fires was at least 140 parts per million, and that it usually approached 1,000 parts per million. So what Dr. Lynch found in the ashes was perfectly consistent with what was to be expected. If Professor Bone was correct his evidence destroyed one of the prosecution's main props. But when Mr. Caswell included it in Charlotte's appeal it was rejected on the grounds that the evidence against her was over-whelming.

She appeared to take the news quietly, but her hair turned white while she awaited the executioner. She was hanged on Wednesday, July 15th, 1936, while a few miles away Leonard Parsons was having drinks with some mates in a village pub.

The poison chosen by Richard Brinkley of Fulham, in an attempt to kill his friend Reginald Parker – an accountant's clerk who lived in lodgings in Croydon – was prussic acid. Brinkley wanted Parker out of the way because the accountant's clerk knew he had falsified a signature on a will. The will was that of an elderly woman who had herself died in mysterious circumstances within a few days of signing over all her worldly goods to Brinkley. Instead of Parker drinking the bottle of poisoned stout that Brinkley offered him, it was mistakenly drunk by Parker's landlord and landlady, Richard and Daisy Beck, and by their daughter Daisy.

There are few poisons which are so ruthlessly efficient as prussic acid and its derivative, cyanide of potassium. Taken in solution on an empty stomach it often kills in a few seconds, like a fatal stroke of lightning and in exactly the same way – by paralysis of the breathing. Within minutes Mr. and Mrs. Beck and their daughter were writhing on the floor. Another daughter hastily summoned a doctor, but by the time he arrived all Mr. and Mrs. Beck were dead. The daughter survived.

Brinkley was arrested and claimed in his defence that he had not wanted to kill the Becks – he only wanted to kill Reginald Parker, and had failed. It turned out that he had something of a reputation in the poisons business. Some years previously a neighbour had found Mrs. Brinkley dead on a sofa, and had called the police. They found an opened case of bottles containing prussic acid, strychnine, arsenic, ergot of rye, and chloroform in Brinkley's study. Mrs. Brinkley had died of arsenic poisoning, and with no proof to link her death to her husband a coroner's jury returned a verdict of suicide. Shortly after that Brinkley befriended 17-year-old Laura Glenn, who subsequently died of arsenical poisoning in his rented room in Chelsea. No one has ever suggested she was murdered – indeed, she left a suicide note. Even so, Laura's name has to be added to the impressive list of women who once they got to know Richard Brinkley didn't live for very much longer.

For the murder of the Becks, Richard Brinkley was sentenced to hang. No one will ever know how many people he poisoned, but as the noose tightened around his neck on the scaffold of Wandsworth Prison on Tuesday, August 13th, 1907, he was still trying to convince everyone that he hadn't killed anyone at all.

12

DNA–THE NEW WONDER DETECTION KIT

*He was determined to get rid of the body. He
buried it, dug it up again, reburied it in concrete,
then dug up the concrete, burned the body and
reburied the ashes*

Some of the cases in this book will have
demonstrated that the advancement of forensic
knowledge over the past fifty years has been so rapid
that the chances of murderers and other serious
criminals beating the medical evidence are now very
poor indeed. In the early 1980s a new discovery was
revealed that will reduce those chances even more.
This was the development of DNA (deoxyribonucleic
acid) profiling.

Much earlier in the century forensic scientists had
discovered a method of determining a person's blood
group from their semen or saliva; as a result it became
a matter of routine to preserve a rapist's semen stains.
But proving a criminal's blood group is a long way
from proving his guilt. Then came two important
discoveries: first, that DNA, found in every one of the
cells that go into the making of a human being, was
the magic building-block of life, determining the
genetic characteristics we get handed down from our
parents, and second, that each cell can be analysed
and a DNA profile obtained.

"The blueprint for life" – all the information
required to create a human being – is contained within

the DNA in a human body. This information is carried in the chromosomes which are found in the nuclei of all human cells. Each cell contains 46 chromosomes, 23 from the father's sperm and 23 from the mother's ovum, and each one contains encoded information in the form of DNA arranged in groups of genes.

Until the development of DNA profiling, scientific techniques were used to identify the origin of blood and tissue samples, but there were limitations: if the samples had deteriorated, or if there was not enough material, the forensic scientist could never be sure of accuracy. The discovery that made DNA a method of positive identification of any person from the smallest trace of their body fluid or tissue was made by Professor Alec Jeffreys in 1984. He found that within the DNA molecule of a person was information which was unique to that person, as unique as a fingerprint, giving rise to the term "DNA fingerprinting." Even a tiny amount of blood or semen or a hair found at the scene of a serious crime could be analysed and a DNA profile obtained which could be compared with the profile of a suspect. If there was a match, the identification could be regarded as positive.

The first use of Dr. Jeffreys' discovery in a criminal case came in November, 1987, when Robert Melias burgled a house in Bristol and raped the woman occupier. Melias was picked out on an identity parade, and semen stains from the victim's clothing were compared with his blood sample – the match was perfect. Melias got eight years for rape and five years for robbery. It was now only a question of time before DNA profiling was used for the first time in a murder case. One such case was already to hand in Enderby, in Leicester, where just before the trial of Robert Melias the body of Dawn Ashworth, 15, battered to death and raped, had been found near a lonely footpath. Detectives leading the murder hunt were certain that there were essential similarities between the murder and rape of Dawn and the murder and rape three years earlier of another 15-year-old, Lynda Mann. As had become usual, the rapist's semen was preserved, but the killer left no other clues in either of the two cases.

But now that Dr. Jeffreys' DNA fingerprinting technique was perfected it would be sufficient to obtain a positive comparison of the killer's blood sample with the semen found at the crime scene to secure a conviction. So, certain that the murderer was a local man, police asked for all the young men in Enderby and surrounding villages to give a blood sample. There were 5,000 of them, and when the samples were analysed and compared with the stored semen the killer was not among them.

While the police, completely baffled, were wondering what to do next a young man named Ian Kelly was heard bragging in a Leicester pub about how he had been paid £200 to give a blood sample to the police in place of a friend, who had asked to be helped out. The conversation was reported to the police and Kelly was arrested. He soon confessed that the friend he had aided was Colin Pitchfork, 27, who lived in one of the villages where blood samples had been taken. Pitchfork had apparently panicked and enlisted the aid of his friend when the blood-sample request was made, because he had two previous convictions for indecent exposure and imagined that he would be a prime suspect. For the £200 payment Kelly had not only given his own blood but had claimed he was actually Pitchfork, and had forged Pitchfork's signature.

Colin Pitchfork, a married man, was arrested and the DNA from his blood sample proved to be identical with the DNA samples extracted from the semen at the scenes of the double rape and murder. On both occasions, he confessed, he went out looking for a girl to expose himself to, and when both times he found the girl was alone he was led to rape and murder. He was sentenced at Leicester Crown Court to life for both murders, with 10 years concurrently for the rapes, three years for two additional cases of indecent assault, and three years for conspiracy to pervert the course of justice.

As sensational perhaps as Pitchfork's conviction was the revelation that before his arrest the police had charged a 17 year-old youth with the murder of Dawn Ashworth, and were therefore convinced that the murder hunt was over. But DNA genetic fingerprinting proved that the teenager was not the killer. What would have happened, one wonders, if the new technique had not been in place to prove that he was innocent?

A year after the Pitchfork trial another married man was found guilty of murder as a result of genetic fingerprinting. He was Ian Simms, landlord of the George and Dragon pub at Billinge, St. Helens, Lancashire. His 22-year-old victim, Helen McCourt, disappeared on the afternoon of Tuesday, February 9th, 1988, and when her anxious parents went to the police detectives set to work to reconstruct her last movements. They discovered that she left her office at the Liverpool Royal Insurance Company at 4 p.m., and caught the 4.16 train from Liverpool Lime Street to St. Helens. At St. Helens station she boarded a bus for Billinge, where she lived. The driver remembered her getting off the bus at 5.15 p.m. She then had only a couple of hundred yards to walk to her parents' house.

In the drawer of her office desk police found her diary. There were a number of references in it to Ian Simms, the local publican and the father of two children. They questioned everyone along Billinge High Street, where the pub was situated. A woman told them she remembered a scream, sharp and high-pitched, coming from the vicinity of the pub soon after Helen got off the bus.

Helen, it seemed, was well known at the George and Dragon. She drank there regularly, staying long after closing time, sometimes until early morning. But two days before she disappeared Simms barred her from the premises.

Questioned by detectives, Simms emerged as a man who held matrimony in some disdain. His mistress lived in a flat above the pub, and his wife Nadine and their children lived in a house a few hundred yards away. On the evening of Helen's disappearance, he said, he had been with his mistress, and had not left the pub. But as he spoke he twitched nervously, stuttering over his words. Convinced he was hiding something, the detectives took him to the police station for further questioning. They also questioned his mistress.

At the police station an observant interrogator asked him, "How did you get those scratches on your face, Ian?"

"I was out with the dog, walking through brambles and nettles," Simms replied.

Then another detective came into the interview room. "Ian," he said, "your girl friend has told us what happened on the afternoon and evening of Helen's disappearance. She says you didn't come to the pub until ten o'clock. So where were you?"

His face wet with perspiration, Simms nodded his head. "It's true what she says. I was late getting back that evening. I was sitting alone on Southport beach. I was crying. I've been so upset about my marriage – it's falling apart. I should have mentioned it before, but I was too ashamed."

A suspect who has his alibi shot down, then cannot account for his movements, is a suspect indeed. By this time detectives had searched Simms's car and found an earring with its clip missing. The earring was identified as Helen's by her mother, who said Helen had been wearing it on the day of her disappearance. Asked what he knew about it, Simms shook his head and said, "I haven't seen Helen since Sunday. Someone must have put it in my car."

Warming to the trail, the police called in a forensic scientist, Dr. John Moore, who found bloodstains in the boot of Simms' car. In the bedroom of the flat above the pub detectives found the missing earring clip. They also found tiny tufts of human hair, some of it torn out by the roots, near the bed. There was human blood on Simms' sweat-shirt, human blood on the stairs and floor. Pub staff testified that they had seen Simms scrubbing the floor; his explanation was that his dog had made a mess. They also noticed a lot of plastic bin-liners were gone from the cupboard. There were circumstances here that suggested beyond doubt that Helen had been in the flat, and had come to a violent end.

But one thing was missing. The body. Once there would not have been much of a case without it. But after Dr. Jeffreys' DNA discovery it was of less importance.

The blood on Simms' clothes was undoubtedly human, but was it Helen's? There was now a sure way to find out. Forensic scientists took blood samples from Helen's mother and father, and carried out a DNA genetic fingerprinting test to determine their code. Then they compared it with the blood found on Simms's clothes. The result was that the blood on the clothes was 126,000 times more likely to have come from an offspring of Mr. and Mrs. McCourt than from a randomly selected member of the population.

Once again detectives asked Simms about the scratch-marks on his face and neck. Again he changed his story. His wife had attacked him, he said, after finding out about his affair. But when his wife was questioned she said she knew nothing about his affair until the police told her.

Simms had been in custody for nearly three weeks when a jogger found Helen's handbag beside the River Irwell, 15 miles from Billinge. A search of the area revealed a man's bloodstained jeans, a bloodstained towel and a pair of boots dumped on a slag-heap. They belonged to Ian Simms.

Simms refused to recognise the clothing when shown it by the police. He said, "I have felt in recent weeks that someone has been in the flat with their own set of keys. Someone could have taken my clothes and driven my car away."

That, Merseyside police decided, was enough. Simms was put on trial on Tuesday, February 21st, 1989, at Liverpool Crown Court. Mr. Brian Leveson QC, prosecuting, told the jury that forensic science would prove beyond all doubt that Helen was murdered by the man in the dock. "Her body has been hidden so well that it has not been found, although a very considerable effort has been put into looking for it," he said.

An unusual pale-coloured mud had been found on a bracelet and two rings Simms had been wearing when he was arrested. That mud did not come from Southport beach. The mud was very similar to that found on his clothing and in his car. This meant that Simms had "at least been up to his wrists in pale mud."

Helen's mother told the court that there was one occasion in September, 1987, when Helen stayed out all night, not returning home until 8 a.m. The entry in Helen's diary for that date confirmed that she had spent the night at the George and Dragon. Another entry referred to a night when Helen stayed out until 4 a.m. The inference was that Helen and Ian Simms had been lovers. Mrs. McCourt knew nothing about her daughter being barred from the pub.

Simms's mistress said she was 18 when she first had sex with him, towards the end of 1986. A few months later she started sleeping at the pub. Simms, she said, was sleeping permanently at the pub, telling his wife it was for "security reasons."

She and Simms went on holiday together to Tenerife and toured Britain, staying at the best hotels. During her evidence she cried out, "I loved him, and I still do." Then she broke down.

Cross-examined, she said she had often seen Helen McCourt at the pub. Helen was one of the regular "stay behinds." A couple of days before Helen vanished she heard there had been an argument in the pub between Helen and another girl. Simms had to split them up. The girlfriend said that on the night in question Simms called her and told her not to come to the pub before 8.30 p.m. He did not actually arrive until about 10 p.m. He explained his lateness by saying that his wife had found out about their affair and got into a temper. He pointed to his neck and said, "Look what she's done." There were two faint red marks a couple of inches long. She then went down to look after the bar while Simms took a bath. The next night she found out about Helen's disappearance. She went to the pub and talked to Simms about it while he was working on his account books.

The man who found Simms' bloodstained clothing on the canal towpath said that a few minutes earlier he had seen a car close to the canal bank. "The jeans were muddy and the clay was wet. I put my hand over the top of them by the crotch and it seemed warm to me. I thought they had been dumped there a few minutes before I arrived."

A police surgeon, Dr. Miles Clarke, examined Simms after his arrest and found numerous fine scratches on his body, legs and arms. Some of these were consistent with having been caused by fingernails, others by vegetation.

Simms, giving evidence on his own behalf, said he had once been to bed with Helen – apart from that they were merely good friends. Asked about a bloody fingerprint found on the door at the bottom of the stairs leading to the flat above the pub, he said it had been there for two months. A lot of people had been in and out of the pub, particularly on New Year's Eve.

"I had not seen Helen since the Monday night," he said. "I have never set eyes on her. I never touched her."

Why, he was asked, did a knot in the electrical flex, which was found with Helen's clothes, contain hair matching Helen's? Simms thought someone must have managed to get the flex and put her hair in the knot, in order to "fix him up." None of this convinced the jury, who returned with a guilty verdict. After Simms was sentenced to life imprisonment he continued to stick to his story. Shouting, "I've never seen the girl!" he was hustled from the dock.

Helen McCourt was undoubtedly murdered by Simms, whose concealment of her body has been so complete that it has not been found to this day. But in strict legal terms the body was unnecessary – just her hair and a few bloodstains were all that were needed to catch her killer with DNA genetic fingerprinting.

Interestingly, while genetic fingerprinting has become quickly adopted in Britain as a means of linking murderers to their crimes, courts in the United States, while gradually accepting it, have shown more caution over it. The first time it was used in the state of Virginia concerned a serial killer known as the Southside Slayer at large in Richmond.

The Slayer's victims were white women who he assaulted while they were asleep. He left few clues and no witnesses. He was caught only because the new identification tool traced him through his genetic make-up.

The Slayer struck first on September 17th, 1987, when, investigating an abandoned car outside a block of flats, a police officer discovered 35-year-old Debbie Davis sprawled on the bed in her apartment. She was naked; her hands were tied behind her back and the bonds were wrapped around her neck. Detectives deduced that she was sound asleep when the intruder entered the flat through a kitchen window. Ripping off her nightdress, he tied her hands with rope, raped her and started to strangle her. Then he tied her tights around her neck, looping them through the rope that bound her hands behind her back, in such a way that the slightest movement caused the noose to tighten. He left her to suffer a slow, agonising death.

More murders in Richmond followed over the weeks to come. The next victim was 32-year-old Dr. Susan Hellams, a neurosurgeon. She had gone to bed, and had been tied up, raped and strangled by her attacker. Seven weeks later a 15-year-old student, Diane Cho, was found bound and naked in her bedroom. She had been sexually assaulted and strangled. Two months after that Richmond police got their first real lead. It came from Arlington, Virginia, where local police were seeking information about a 25-year-old convicted burglar arrested on a rape-murder charge. The victim in this case was 44-year-old Susan Tucker, who had been dead in bed for a week when police found her. Her nude body lay face down on the bed with a sleeping bag thrown over it. She had been raped and sodomised by an intruder who had broken in through a bathroom window.

The crime was so neat, with so few things undisturbed, that it reminded an Arlington detective of a burglar he had once put away. The man's name was Timothy Spencer, who in September, 1984, had been transferred to a Richmond "halfway house" – an institution where paroled prisoners in America live before their release. He had a string of convictions for burglary, but no sex-offence convictions.

At the halfway house police found a camouflage jacket belonging to Spencer which contained fragments of glass that matched the distinctive glass of the broken window in Susan Tucker's home. Spencer was asked to give a blood sample. Tested in New York, it showed that the genetic material in his blood was identical to that in dried semen scraped from Susan Tucker's thigh. The scientists who made the test said the chances of two people having the same genetic make-up was about 135 million to one. While Spencer was locked up on charges of sexual assault and murder his genetic profile turned up in body fluids discovered at the crime scenes in the Debbie Davis and Susan Hellams cases. Although he was the prime suspect in the murder of Diane Cho, he could not be charged because not enough semen had been recovered to conduct DNA testing.

Spencer, linked to nine other rape cases, was put on trial for the murder of Susan Tucker in Virginia's first ever case that was to stand or fall on the evidence of genetic profiling. The technique was so new that Prosecutor Arthur Karp called six scientists to testify about its reliability and its use in six other states.

The experts emphasised that the DNA test could not yield a false positive result which would incorrectly identify a suspect. "One could get a false negative from not being careful," one scientist said. "But I can't think of a way you can get a false positive from not being careful." Only a sibling could have the same DNA make-up as its parents, it was explained.

The jury were told that after the police found Susan Tucker's body, a cloth underneath it, a sleeping-bag that partially covered her, and a nightgown lying next to her were taken for DNA testing. All three items were semen-stained, and were tested against a sample of Spencer's blood. The stains were identical to the sample.

A photograph showing DNA patterns of semen stains next to the DNA patterns of the defendant's blood was enlarged on an overhead projector and shown to the jury on a big screen. Using a yardstick, a DNA forensic scientist pointed three times to corresponding patterns of dots on the screen. "Nightgown, sleeping-bag, defendant's blood," she recited. "Nightgown, sleeping-bag, defendant's blood. Nightgown, sleeping-bag, defendant's blood."

Defence attorney Carl Womack tried an unusual method in an attempt to break down the prosecution's case. He did not dispute the findings, but questioned the scientist closely about the chance that blood relatives could have the same DNA patterns. Then he called the defendant's relatives and asked each of them to list the names of family members. The strategy was to show that relatives living in Arlington had the same genetic make-up as the defendant, and that therefore any of them could have been capable of committing the murders.

Prosecutor Karp objected loudly. With the jury absent, he contended that if the defence was allowed to continue with this argument he should be allowed to introduce DNA and other evidence linking Spencer to the rape and murder of Susan Hellams and Debbie Davis. In addition to the DNA testing, Mr. Karp said, Spencer was linked to the crimes by more than a dozen similarities, among them that the victims were white women living alone; each victim's hands were tied behind her back; in two cases a rope ran from their bound hands to around their necks; each was strangled; each lived within walking distance of where Spencer was staying when the murders occurred; all were killed at a time when Spencer was signed out from his parole residence; no money was found in the victims' handbags; the blood type belonging to the suspect in all three cases was identical to Spencer's; and a window was broken to gain entrance.

Judge Benjamin Kendrick agreed with the prosecutor. He told defence lawyer Womack that if he continued with the strategy that suggested that a relative could have murdered Susan Tucker he would allow the prosecutor to introduce evidence from other murders. "I think you've opened up the door, and no matter what you do, you can't have your cake and eat it too," the judge said.

After an hour of discussion lawyers on both sides agreed to a stipulation that none of Spencer's relatives had committed the crime. They also agreed to omit the Richmond evidence from the trial and drop the issue of blood relatives as suspects. The next day Spencer gave evidence on his own behalf, insisting that he did not rape or murder Susan Tucker. He asserted that he had never even seen or heard of her before his arrest. The jurors found that difficult to believe, and on July 17th they found him guilty of first-degree rape and murder. They determined that he should go to prison for life. As the verdict was read the slight, slow-talking defendant sat impassively clutching his mother's hand.

Back in Britain, where DNA genetic fingerprinting was discovered, the new technique continued to chalk up successes. One noteworthy case occurred in Swansea in 1994 when a drug-dealer, Danny Dyke, mysteriously disappeared.

Dyke lived a double life. His apparently respectable

existence as an osteopath was a cover for his extensive dealings in the world of illegal drugs – he was a middle-man between major drug dealers in London and wholesale customers in Swansea and other parts of South Wales. His respectable side included being a physiotherapist for Aberavon Rugby Club in the 1992-93 season; his less than respectable side was that he was supplying cannabis, amphetamines and Ecstasy to a network of contacts.

Police began an investigation in the spring of 1994 largely because of drug-dealing rumours sweeping through Swansea. When Danny Dyke's Ford Escort R. S. Turbo car was found abandoned in suspicious circumstances, they decided to act, arresting John Welsby and John Wilson, who were both involved in the drugs scene.

One of the rumours suggested that Danny Dyke had been killed after a fight in the kitchen of John Wilson's semi-detached house in Elba Crescent, Crymlyn Burrows, on Wednesday, April 13th, 1994. When detectives went to investigate they found that the kitchen had been almost entirely renewed – new cabinets, new floor, even new wall tiles, and the whole place had been steam-cleaned. Nevertheless, forensic scientists set to work to try to extract some evidence, such as a bloodstain, from this massive clean-up operation.

They were getting nowhere when a workman came by. He said he had been instructed by John Wilson to change the kitchen doors, and was now calling for his money. The original doors, he said, were still in his garage. More confident that there might be some clues after all, Clair Galbraith, of the forensic science team, went to examine the doors.

"I found a number of minute bloodspots," she reported. "The pattern of them was interesting because it was typical of that resulting from a blow into wet blood – a blow caused by someone who is hitting someone who is bleeding. I marked them on a sketchplan, then lifted them for DNA analysis."

The bloodstains were so minute that they had to be multiplied many times, a process known as DNA amplification. The sample is put into nutriment and allowed to grow. The larger sample is then mixed with a jelly that conducts electricity. As the current passes through the DNA it leaves a distinct trace – the DNA profile for that individual. The trace was compared with a sample of blood from Mr. and Mrs. Dyke, the parents of Danny, and it was a positive match. All that this proved, though, was that Danny Dyke must have been at Elba Crescent and that he was beaten up. There were a number of other bloodstains on the bottom of the kitchen door, but when tested they did not match the profile of anyone involved in the case. Wilson's wife told the police that there had been a fight, and the kitchen was a mess.

John Welsby, who was due to be sentenced at Swansea Crown Court for various offences concerning his role as a "money-taker" in drug trafficking, suggested a deal to Chief Superintendent Phil Jones, head of South Wales CID. "Give me fifty grand and get me off my charge," he said, "and I'll show you where Danny Dyke's body is."

That, of course, isn't the kind of arrangement in which the police can co-operate, but some sort of a compromise was reached, and Welsby made an extraordinary statement. He said he knew that Danny Dyke was coming down from London for a rendezvous at John Wilson's house in Elba Crescent to drop off some drugs and collect payment. On the afternoon of April 13th Welsby received a phone call from Wilson telling him to come quickly, and to bring a van. Welsby went with his brother Terry to Elba Crescent, where they found Dyke dead on the kitchen floor, blood all over the room and John Wilson in a state of panic.

Welsby's story was that he and his brother Terry bundled the body, wrapped in a carpet from Wilson's kitchen, into the van, leaving Wilson to clean up the mess in the kitchen. They decided to bury it in the same land at Garnswilt, near Ammanford, that John Welsby sometimes used for tipping. But several weeks later John Welsby began to get nervous about the grave. He had heard rumours that people were poaching and digging for badgers on the site, and climbing a hill that overlooked it. If a dog sniffed out the body ...

So, obsessed by the idea that someone would find the body, he dug it up again and re-buried it in concrete, and then, days later, he dug up the concrete, extracted the body, burned it, and reburied the ashes.

When Chief Superintendent Jones was listening to this astonishing story he might have had reason to regard it as another one of the red herrings that Welsby liked to lay around his criminal career, but this time he believed him. Welsby took police officers to the piece of land and paced out the grave. When the police returned four days later to start digging they brought with them an archaeologist, and forensic scientist John Owen.

This was to be no ordinary exhumation, because everyone knew that Welsby had set out to destroy the body completely. All they could do was look for forensic clues. The search for anything that would link the site with what had happened in Wilson's kitchen was hampered by a turn in the weather that brought snow and bitingly cold wind. A mechanical digger made no impact on the rock-hard ground, so it was down to pick-axes and shovels.

After some back-breaking work the diggers came across some bits of burned concrete. One piece contained a fragment of blue fabric. The police knew there had been a blue carpet in Wilson's kitchen, and that it had been used to wrap the body. The fabric was taken to a forensic laboratory where it was tested for blood. The technique used is to rub the piece of fabric with filter paper, then to test the filter paper chemically. If there is blood present, the chemicals turn green. The result was positive – blood was present on the fabric.

Could it be proved to be part of the carpet from Wilson's house? The police checked up on carpet retailers and found the one who sold the carpet to Wilson. They also learned from him about another customer who had bought exactly the same kind of carpet. The fabric from the waste land was then compared microscopically with the other customer's carpet – they were identical.

As they went deeper the archaeologist began to identify scorch marks in the hole they were digging. It was clear that the fire must have been intense – they could only hope to find some piece that somehow had escaped the inferno. And their patience was rewarded. What appeared to be a tiny fragment of bone was lifted out on a spade and examined by the archaeologist. It was a piece of human skull, and DNA profiling identified it with Danny Dyke.

All through his explanations of what had happened, John Welsby had insisted that his brother Terry was not implicated in the case. Now, working on a hunch, Swansea police decided to take a blood sample from Terry Welsby and to compare it with the unidentified bloodstains on Wilson's discarded kitchen doors. The DNA was an exact match.

Terry Welsby's answer to this revealing forensic evidence was to say that he had done some building work in Wilson's kitchen and had injured himself, drawing blood. But that version of events wasn't accepted by the police. John Welsby and John Wilson were charged with murder.

Both blamed each other for the attack on Danny Dyke. John Welsby said he had given £16,000 to Dyke when they met earlier that fatal day at a house in Rhondda Street, Swansea. From Rhondda Street Dyke went to see Wilson at Elba Crescent. When Welsby himself later went to Wilson's house at Elba Crescent he said he found Dyke had been beaten with a hammer and throttled with a kettle lead by Wilson.

Wilson's account was that his house was being used for a drugs-related business meeting between Welsby and Dyke. He claimed he had never seen Dyke before Welsby brought him for the meeting at about 6 p.m. Wilson said he went upstairs while Welsby and Dyke went into the kitchen. When he heard noises he came downstairs to find them fighting. He intervened and pushed Dyke back against some cupboards, and at that point he saw that Dyke had two serious facial injuries.

Dyke ducked down as Welsby again went for him with a hammer. The blow came into contact with Wilson's head and nearly knocked him out. As he fell to his knees he heard another noise and saw that Dyke was also on the floor, breathing heavily. When Terry Welsby arrived, said Wilson, Dyke was in a pool of blood on the kitchen carpet and was spitting violently. After the two brothers got Dyke into a standing position they took him out to the van. Wilson claimed that Dyke must have been killed later somewhere else, because when the drugs-dealer left Elba Crescent he was still on his feet.

The jury took nearly 14 hours to find Wilson and John Welsby guilty of murder. They were given life sentences, and Terry Welsby, charged with perverting the course of justice, got thirty months.

No one knows exactly what the killing of Danny

Dyke was about. But a fair surmise is that when he arrived at Wilson's house from London with his stash of drugs that April 13th, John Welsby and John Wilson were waiting for him. There was a row – perhaps because Dyke had been double-dealing. He was beaten to death, and his body was taken off for its first burial on the Garnswilt waste land. The rest was done by DNA profiling – surely one of the greatest discoveries in forensic medicine's spectacular war on crime.